A Textbook of Den

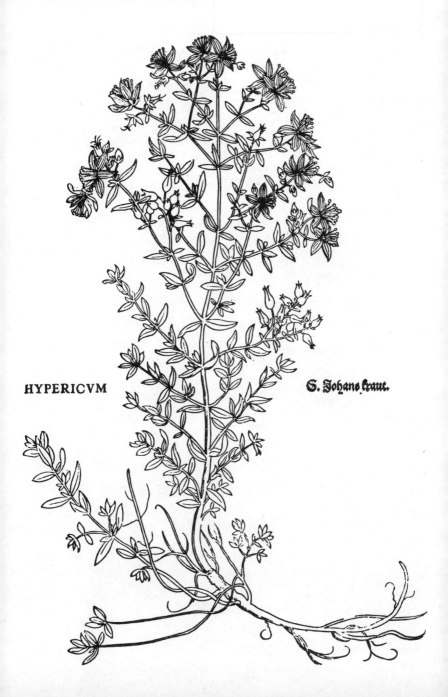

HYPERICVM

S. Johans kraut.

A Textbook of Dental Homoeopathy

for dental surgeons, homoeopathists and general medical practitioners
by
Dr Colin B. Lessell
MB, BS (Lond), BDS (Lond), MRCS (Eng), LRCP (Lond)
Vice-Chairman British Homoeopathic Dental Association

With an appendix on mercury toxicity by
Catherine Price

Index compiled by
Lyn Greenwood

Illustrated

Saffron Walden
The C.W. Daniel Company Limited

First published in Great Britain in 1995
by The C.W. Daniel Company Limited
1 Church Path, Saffron Walden
Essex, CB10 1JP, England

ISBN 0 85207 281 3

This book is printed on part-recycled paper

Produced by Book Production Consultants plc
Designed and Typeset by Cambridge Photosetting Services
Printed and bound by St Edmundsbury Press, Bury St Edmunds, Suffolk

To Dr Richard Fischer, DDS
and my other American colleagues

'Do not talk of colour to the blind'
Turkish proverb

Contents

Illustrations List

Introduction

This concise work is primarily intended for the use of the dental profession, including students and specialists in its various fields. Nevertheless, the professional homoeopathist and the homoeopathically inclined general medical practitioner will also find it a useful source of reference in practice where he or she is confronted with a patient presenting with an orofacial condition. The book is divided into two major parts, supplemented by two appendices.

PART ONE is a basic introduction to the principles of homoeopathic pharmacy and prescribing, especially directed towards newcomers. Though fairly simple in its content, it does contain a more advanced approach to dental homoeopathic teaching, whereby general and psychological characteristics of the patient are considered to be determinants for a prescription based on the presenting complaint itself.

PART TWO is an encyclopaedic section. Alphabetically arranged and thoroughly cross-referenced, it is a combined materia medica and therapeutic index of homoeopathic treatments. Moreover, it also constitutes a self-tuition course in dental homoeopathy. Peter Galgut is to be thanked for allowing me to utilise his ideas on homoeopathic periodontology. Important aspects of nutrition, and the value of certain botanic medicines are subjects also considered.

Appendix One concerns the composition and acquisition of a dental pharmacy for your surgery. *Appendix Two* is an analysis of the current views on mercury toxicity contributed by Catherine Price. Its removal from the main text, and its relegation to an individual appendix, is to emphasise its importance and relevance.

This present work thus differs considerably in content and size from my original concise work 'The Dental Prescriber'. The development of the text has been assisted by the valuable contributions of Richard Fischer of the USA and the clinical work of the members of the British Homoeopathic Dental Association (BHDA), created some four years ago by a small band of enthusiasts, and whose membership has now grown considerably.

The BHDA now runs annual courses on dental homoeopathy, in conjunction with those of the Royal London Homoeopathic Hospital. Those who are interested should contact the Department of Research and Education, The Royal London Homoeopathic Hospital, Great Ormond Street, London WC1N 3HR (Tel: 0171 837 8833; Fax: 0171 833 7269). They will also supply you with the current mailing address and telephone number of the Secretary of the BHDA, from whom further details of that organisation may be obtained. In the USA, the BHDA representative is Dr Richard Fischer, DDS, 4222 Evergreen Lane, Annandale, Virginia 22003, to whom you may write.

Examinations in dental homoeopathy have recently been established, for which the content of the present book will be adequate for supplying the purely dental requirements.

Dr C B Lessell

MB, BS, BDS, MRCS, LRCP

PART ONE

Homoeopathy in a Nutshell

What is homoeopathy?

Homoeopathy may be defined as that school of medicine founded by Dr [Christian Friedrich] Samuel Hahnemann, the medicinal therapeusis of which differs markedly from that of orthodox medicine, or *allopathy*, as it is termed.

Who was Hahnemann?

Samuel Hahnemann, born at Meissen in Germany in 1755, was a physician, polyglottic translator and medical reformer. Appalled by the illogical and often harmful orthodox medical practices of the day, he sought to discover better and safer ways of prescribing medicines. His first major work on homoeopathic ideology, the *Organon*, was published in 1810. The sixth and final edition of this book, however, although completed a year or so before his death in Paris in 1843, remained unpublished until 1921.

What is Hahnemann's fundamental proposition?

Hahnemann's fundamental proposition, now peculiar to homoeopathy, may be expressed thus:

'That the selection of a drug to treat a particular disease in the sick individual should be determined by its ability to induce a *similar* disease in the *healthy*.'

This proposition is termed the *Law of Similars*, more concisely expressed in Latin as *Similia similibus curentur* ('Let likes be treated with likes'). The implication of this 'law' is that lesser doses have the opposite effect of greater.

Whereas other authors, including Hippocrates, had suggested the occasional use of drugs upon an analogous basis, it was for Hahnemann to transform his proposition into the foundation for an extensive and valuable therapeutic system, which we term *homoeopathy*.

Toxicity & the Law of Similars

An important aspect of the Law of Similars, which has been established empirically, is that it continues to hold true even as the material therapeutic dose is considerably reduced. This matter is highly significant with regard to essentially toxic materials, such as mercury, where sub-toxic dosages may still exert a curative effect.

An example of the application of the Law of Similars

The symptoms of mercury poisoning include halitosis, gingivitis and periodontitis. In accordance with the Law of Similars, homoeopathically prepared *Mercurius solubilis*, given in non-toxic quantities, may be used to treat some (but not all) types of gingival and periodontal disease. We shall say more of homoeopathic pharmaceutical technique later, but, for the moment, note that the homoeopathic version of the drug is generally expressed in a *latinized* form (with few exceptions), in accordance with established international custom.

More about cause & cure

The picture of *disease* induced by the action of a drug is termed its *pathogenesis*. It includes both psychological and physical objective and subjective symptoms, and pathological and physiological changes. The pathogenesis is established by recording the effects generated by the drug when it is administered either accidentally or intentionally. An important type of intentional administration is the so-called homoeopathic *experimental proving*, where a drug is administered to a number of *healthy* human volunteers who subsequently document the changes experienced; for which purpose, the drug is administered either in a crude form or as an attenuated homoeopathic preparation ('sporadic proving' may also occur during actual treatment, when the patient generates new and unusual symptoms related to the medicine given). The results of *provings* (experimental and sporadic), together with the symptomatic and pathological details recorded in cases of accidental or malicious poisoning (*toxicology*), constitute the basis of the homoeopathic *materia medica*. When you read about symptoms or diseases in works of homoeopathic materia medica, you must realise that it is implied that the relevant drug may either *cause* or *cure* the listed abnormalities, according to circumstances and dosage. Further on we shall examine the structure of the materia medica, and discuss how it has been (and *is being*) modified and amplified in the light of *clinical experience*.

What is the simillimum?

The closer the similarity between the documented pathogenesis of a drug and the disease picture of a particular patient, the more likely will that drug effect a cure in that patient. Drugs which exhibit such a close correspondence are said to be *homoeopathic* to the disease. The drug which is felt to have the greatest symptomatic and pathological correspondence is termed the *simillimum* ('most similar'), a more expansive definition of which shall be provided later in the text. For the moment, let it be emphasised that the selection of the simillimum rests not only upon the orthodox diagnostic entity (the name of the disease) but, in many instances, also upon the individualised objective and subjective symptomatology. Such symptomatic pictures may vary considerably between cases of disease within the same conventional diagnostic category (e.g. influenza), each case requiring a different simillimum. In other situations (such as *acute dental abscess*) the symptomatic response is more uniform, and thus the choice of a possible simillimum more limited, and hence simpler.

When is a drug not a drug?

Shortly we shall be discussing homoeopathic pharmaceutical preparation, one objective of which is the attenuation of toxicity of potentially harmful drugs. By definition, a *drug* is any substance used for its medicinal action, be it current or obsolete; a term which, therefore, might even include attenuated homoeopathic preparations. However, common parlance supports our brief that homoeopathic attenuations should be termed *remedies* rather than *drugs*, the implication being that they are less noxious and immensely safer. Some, however, prefer to call them *medicines*, again implying something more benign.

From which classes of substance are homoeopathic remedies derived?

Contrary to popular notion, which confuses homoeopathy with herbalism, homoeopathic remedies are not solely derived from the vegetable kingdom. Many are prepared from minerals, and some from animal products, such as snake venoms. Between the animal and the vegetable kingdom, bacteria, viruses, protozoa and microfungi (or the tissues and exudates containing them) are transformed into remedies of great therapeutic importance, termed *nosodes*; a designation which also includes any remedy made from diseased but uninfected tissue (as in cataract, osteoarthrosis or carcinoma). Indeed, one might say that virtually any matter or energetic radiation in the Universe might become a remedy, were its pathogenesis and therapeusis fully established. Even orthodox drugs have been used to create remedies. Perhaps more remarkably, homoeopathic pharmaceutical techniques can also unmask the therapeutic potential of apparently inert substances (such as flint, yielding *Silicea*), the pathogenesis of which can only be established in their homoeopathically prepared form.

What is the objective of homoeopathic pharmaceutical technique?

This objective is twofold:
(1) The attenuation of chemical toxicity.
(2) The preservation, enhancement or development of medicinal action.

What are the stages of homoeopathic pharmaceutical technique?

There are three to be described:
(1) Selection and initial preparation.
(2) Potentisation.
(3) Impregnation.

Selection & initial preparation

Since many homoeopathic remedies are derived from herbaceous plants, it is appropriate that with these the method should be exemplified. Pre-eminently, the plants should be identified as being of the correct species, healthy and vigorous. They should be gathered when in full bloom, and before overt seed formation; preferably on a bright morning after a rainy night. Under such circumstances they will be in their prime, and their pharmacological content generally optimal. Having washed them, the appropriate parts of the plant are selected and finely chopped or minced. Sometimes the whole plant is utilised. In the case of leopard's bane (*Arnica montana*), which yields the important antihaemorrhagic remedy *Arnica*, the root or whole plant may be selected. However, since the flowers may be infested with the Arnica fly, the irritant properties of which resemble those of Spanish fly (urinary tract irritation), it is sometimes preferable to exclude them.

The disrupted material is then *macerated* in ethanol-water in a tightly stoppered glass vessel, in a cool, dark place, and agitated daily. The selected strength of the alcoholic solvent is generally between 60 and 80%, being largely dependent upon the juice content of the plant material. The higher the water content of the material (as assessed by desiccation), the greater the strength of alcohol required. In the case of leopard's bane, eight days of maceration will suffice to ensure adequate *extraction* of the soluble constituents, both organic and mineral.

The contents of the vessel are then decanted, strained and filtered, to yield a liquid which is termed the *mother tincture*, usually denoted by the symbol Ø, or occasionally by the abbreviations *MT* or *TM*. This mother tincture is stored in amber glass bottles in a cool, dark place, and is now ready to be subjected to the next stage of homoeopathic preparation, termed *potentisation*. However, in some cases we may utilise the mother tincture itself for medicinal purposes. *Arnica Ø*, for example, may be applied directly to *unbroken skin* in order to treat bruises and haematomata, but *must not be used in the mouth*, even when mixed with water, because of its irritant properties. Even so, it may infrequently induce an allergic dermatitis (eczema) in some, especially those with sensitive skins. By contrast, *Calendula Ø*, prepared from the marigold *Calendula officinalis*, is perfectly safe as a mouthwash when diluted, and a potent promoter of healing in traumatised soft tissues. Some mother tinctures of extremely low toxicity may be administered internally, as with *Crataegus Ø*, prepared from hawthorn berries and utilised in the treatment of antibiotic-induced diarrhoea.

Mother tinctures can be made from any substance soluble in ethanol-water. These include all manner of plant materials, some minerals (such as phosphorus, for which absolute alcohol is used), and various animal products (such as snake venoms). The preparation of these is delineated in various versions of the *homoeopathic pharmacopoeia*. The trend these days is very much towards one of standardisation of procedure in order to produce international uniformity of quality. Most mother tinctures have a shelf-life of approximately five years, after which time they should be discarded and replaced.

With regard to mother tinctures prepared from plants, a certain amount of toxic attenuation may occur, in that the alcohol denatures certain poisons. In this respect we should cite *Rhus toxicodendron Ø*, prepared from North American poison ivy. Slightest contact with the plant itself induces a terrible herpetiform rash, due to the presence of *urushiol*; yet the mother tincture has no such properties, and is freely incorporated into creams used in the topical treatment of strained ligaments and muscles, and vesicular lesions.

Within the mother tincture, the function of the alcohol is to extract, modify and preserve. The solute which it contains is termed the *original substance*, and how this is *potentised* is the subject of our next discussion.

For the moment, the preparation of substances *insoluble* in ethanol-water will be left in abeyance.

Potentisation

This unique process, peculiar to homoeopathy, consists of *serial dilution* together with the *application of mechanical energy* at each stage. One cannot over-emphasise the fact that it is not merely a matter of simple dilution alone!

Serial dilution implies that each dilution is of equal magnitude and is made from the one that immediately precedes it.

In the case of *Arnica*, one drop of *Arnica Ø* is added to a glass vial containing 99 drops of ethanol-water (strength 15–95%, according to the pharmacy). The vial is stoppered and then violently agitated. This violent mechanical agitation is termed *succussion*, and is more effectively carried out if the vial is not more than three-quarters full. Mechanical succussion devices are available, but the process is very simply carried out manually (for conciseness, the instructions that follow are given for right-handed operators).

Succussion actually consists of two phases: shaking and jolting. The vial is grasped in the palm of the right hand, with the thumb held firmly over the stopper. The vial is shaken well, each shake terminating in a jerk, achieved by striking the closed right hand (which protects the glass) against the open palm of the left hand. This is repeated, according to the custom of the pharmacy, 10–20 times. Rapping the bottom of the vial cautiously on a leather-bound book may be substituted for the use of the left hand. This completes the preparation of the *1st centesimal potency* or *attenuation*, which is labelled *Arnica 1c*. The term *centesimal* refers to the *serial dilution scale* of 1 in 100.

One drop of the 1st centesimal potency or attenuation is then added to 99 drops of ethanol-water in a new vial with a fresh stopper, and this is *succussed* in the same manner as described previously. This yields the *2nd centesimal potency* or *attenuation*, which is labelled *Arnica 2c*. The dilution is now 1 in 10,000 (1 in 10^4).

The processes of serial dilution and succussion continue thereafter in an identical fashion: so, by the time we have prepared *Arnica 30c*, we have thirty stoppered vials, labelled from 1c to 30c, the dilution of the latter being 1 in 10^{60}.

The process of potentisation may be continued almost *ad infinitum*, though normally the highest potency produced is *CM* (=100,000c), corresponding to an extraordinary dilution of 1 in 10^{200000}.

With regard to remedies in general, the most frequently used potencies are 6c, 30c, 200c and M (=1000c). By convention, *the suffix 'c' is often omitted*, so that Arnica 30 = Arnica 30c. Very high potencies, such as 10M (=10,000c), 50M (=50,000c) and CM, are more conveniently prepared by a technique of potentisation known as *Korsakow's method*. Since this method is also useful in the self-preparation of *periodontal nosodes* in dental practice, it is described subsequently.

Later, we shall make mention of two other scales of dilution used in homoeopathy, the *decimal* and the *LM*. The term *liquid potency* is applied to any homoeopathic attenuation in ethanol-water, irrespective of the dilution scale. Such liquid potencies may be administered directly to the patient in the form of drops, a technique particularly useful in the unconscious or semiconscious. More commonly, however, various solid sugars are *impregnated* with them (1 drop per 7–14g), these preparations being more convenient for general use.

Potentisation & medicinal action

One of the great controversies concerning homoeopathic remedies is the issue of their pharmacological effect in extreme dilution. At a dilution of 1 in 10^{12} (potency 6c), the molecular or ionic concentration of an original substance is so small that, in normal clinical dosage, even the most virulent poison is deemed to have negligible chemical toxicity. Furthermore, in dilutions in excess of 1 in 10^{24} (potency 12c) there are no traces of original substance whatsoever (except, perhaps, the odd molecule); hence the concept of the *infinitesimal* dose. However, both clinical and experimental evidence confirm that homoeopathic potencies in excess of 6c, and even 12c, do exhibit predictable pharmacological activity, and that their placebo effect is no greater than might be expected from any medicament, conventional or otherwise. In this respect succussed potencies appear, therefore, to be quite different from unsuccussed simple or serial dilutions.

The usual explanation of this phenomenon is that the act of succussion induces a transfer of 'medicinal energy' from the solute to the diluent; and it is further implied that the diluent is further so energised with each phase of potentisation. Whereas the concept of some sort of energetic transfer is acceptable to many, the rider that suggests a greater energy with dilution, not surprisingly, has met with much disbelief on the part of non-homoeopaths.

The scientific basis of homoeopathy

This rather complex subject is thoroughly discussed in my previous book, *The Infinitesimal Dose*, to which you might wish to refer in due course. However, without going into enormous detail, I will endeavour to summarise the main points.

During succussion, the molecules of the diluent (ethanol and water) are caused to collide with the molecules or ions of the original substance (solute). As a result of collision, there is a transference of energetic quanta (particles), characteristic of the outer electronic energy levels of the donor solute molecule or ion, to the outer (lone pair) electrons of the diluent hydroxyl group (water is effectively a bifurcate hydroxyl group). In this manner, the recipient outer electrons now adopt the same orbital energy levels as those of the donor molecule or ion. This is what might be termed *the inductive chemical imprint*. Such imprinted diluent molecules, during further episodes of succussion, will convey their acquired electronic status to new molecules of diluent by collision; so that, even after the original substance has been diluted out of existence, the electrochemical message is capable of survival and replication.

The application of succussion increases the number of imprinted molecules, but serial dilution must reduce it. However, at each level of serial potentisation (dilution plus succussion), the effect of succussion outweighs that of dilution. Thus, rather as the pilgrim takes two steps forwards and one backwards, the concentration of imprinted diluent molecules edges upwards with further levels of potentisation.

However, succussion also imparts an *oscillatory frequency* to the diluent molecules, which are caused to vibrate in unison. For various reasons, discussed in *The Infinitesimal Dose*, this frequency cannot be increased unless serial dilution always precedes succussion. Higher potencies are associated with higher oscillatory frequencies, but, somewhere around CM (100,000c), the frequency probably becomes maximal.

In summary:

(a) The functions of serial *succussion* are:
   (1) To increase the concentration of imprinted diluent molecules.
   (2) To increase the frequency of oscillation of those molecules.

(b) The functions of serial *dilution* are:
   (1) To remove the original substance (which may be toxic) in stages.
   (2) To slow the increase in concentration of imprinted diluent molecules consequent upon serial succussion.
   (3) To allow the diluent molecules to produce increasing frequencies by means of serial succussion.

What is the significance of 'potency'?

For practical purposes, the term 'oscillatory frequency' may be equated with the term 'potency'. Hence, to talk of a low potency is to refer to a low frequency.

The frequencies manifest by any particular potentised remedy are responsible for the modification of its particular properties. In general, the higher the frequency (and thus the potency number), the more potent are the therapeutic effects of the remedy. It becomes swifter in action and more eradicative of disease; in other words stronger. At the same time, in many cases, its *range* of action is extended, so that profound general physiological and biochemical effects may be experienced throughout the organism, including alterations in the psyche. Such may be termed a *constitutional response*, and the remedy given, a *constitutional remedy*. Not all remedies, however, routinely produce such widespread effects, even in high potency (high frequency). Many, such as *Arnica*, have a more restricted action on the physiology in virtually any potency, and may be described as *pathological remedies*. Lower potencies (e.g. 6c) of so-called constitutional remedies may also manifest such a restricted and pathological action (such as *Pulsatilla* in the treatment of a sty). The type of response (pathological or constitutional) produced by a remedy is also dependent upon patient *sensitivity*; so that sensitive subjects may experience constitutional effects even with low potencies of either type of remedy. Nevertheless, with regard to general and common prescribing in dental practice, whilst one should be aware of this fact, it is seldom a situation that will arise.

What is Korsakow's method of potentisation?

Essentially, this is serial potentisation within a *single* glass vial. Instead of transferring one drop of the liquid potency to another vial of diluent, the vial is emptied, leaving some of the liquid potency adherent to the inner surface. The conformation of the vial is such that approximately one drop remains. To the same vessel, 99 drops (about 3.6ml) of diluent are added, and succussion carried out in the usual way. Again the vial is emptied, more diluent added, and succussion applied. In this way, it is possible to carry out serial potentisation without the need for a large number of vials. In terms of alcohol, however, it is no more economic than the normal method.

This technique is of some limited use in the dental surgery, where we wish to prepare *autonosodes* from gingival material. *Autonosodes* are remedies prepared from infected material, bodily fluids or tissues from an individual, which are then used solely in his or her treatment. In preparing these in the surgery, complying exactly with the centesimal scale is unessential. Any glass vial may be used, as long as it is between 1 and 10ml in size, and is provided with a washable rubber stopper or synthetic cap. A small quantity of gingival exudate, pus or materia alba is gathered with a tiny pledget of cotton-wool. This is placed in the vial, half-filled with

'Polish Pure Spirit', or any other pure form of ethanol, at least 40% in strength. The vial is stoppered, and then succussed. This constitutes the first potency. The vial is then inverted, half-filled with fresh alcohol, and the stopper or cap is washed and dried on a clean cloth. The vial is restoppered and succussion applied, in order to produce the second serial potency. This process is continued up to the 30th level of potentisation. The 6th, 9th, 12th and 30th liquid potencies should be retained and stored in individual labelled amber glass vials for future use (e.g. 'Gingival autonosode #12, Mr D. Egg, 6/6/94). These liquid potencies may be administered directly to the patient, or may be used to impregnate sugar pilules (which are spherical), tablets (which are flat) or granules.

What is the decimal scale?
This is serial potentisation, where the dilution at each stage is 1 in 10, rather than 1 in 100. In order to distinguish them from the centesimal scale preparations, decimal potencies are qualified by the letter 'x', e.g. 6x. It is more popular in Central Europe, where the suffix 'x' is replaced by the prefix 'D'. Hence, D30=30x. However, even in the UK and the USA, the *biochemic tissue salts* and lower potencies of insoluble non-toxic substances (see below) are routinely prepared in this manner.

How are insoluble substances potentised?
Substances which are neither soluble in water or ethanol (such as silica and mercury) are prepared by prolonged *trituration* (grinding) and serial dilution with lactose (milk-sugar), using a ceramic mortar and pestle or some equivalent mechanical device (the inductive chemical imprint of the original substance is probably a function of the lactose hydroxyl groups). The *biochemic tissue salts* are always prepared in this manner. By the time a dilution in lactose of 3c or 6x (both of dilution 1 in 10^6) has been achieved, the original substance will have become colloidally soluble in ethanol-water. Therefore, from 4c or 7x upwards, potentisation proceeds in the liquid phase, as described previously. Below 4c or 7x, the preparations are compressed into tablets. The frequency of any particular numerical potency on the decimal scale tends to be less than that for its numerical equivalent on the centesimal scale. However, for most practical purposes in dentistry, where the centesimal potency (such as 12c) is unavailable, the decimal equivalent (12x or D12) may be substituted and used similarly.

What is the LM scale?

This is rather a specialised scale in homoeopathy, and is of little concern to the beginner. However, you should be aware of its existence, since it grows in popularity amongst homoeopathists. Its fuller name is the *fifty millesimal scale*, since the degree of dilution at each stage is 1 in 50,000. The number of successions applied after each dilution is 100 (rather than 10–20). The scale is a little confusing, however, since LM1 is prepared as a liquid 1 in 50,000 dilution from the 3rd centesimal *trituration* in lactose of either a soluble or insoluble original substance. This is about all you will need to know about it for the time being.

What constitutes a dose?

In general, except in the case of sensitive patients, a remedy may be considered to have a *trigger action*; that is to say, provided a certain minimal dose is given, giving a larger dose will not increase its effect. Generally, an increase in effect can only be produced by giving a higher numerical potency or by repetition of the dose after a particular interval of time. In the oral administration of potentised remedies, which is by far the most common route, a single dose may be taken to be: *one* pilule, tablet or drop. This is the same for both adults and children, with the exception of the *biochemic tissue salts*, where the dose is 4 tables for an adult and 2 for a child. A drop of liquid potency or a small pinch of impregnated fine sugar granules are better suited to the treatment of small children (under 2 years of age), by avoiding the risk of pilule or tablet inhalation. Pilules and fine granules are composed of sucrose, whereas most tables are composed of lactose. In cases of *lactase deficiency*, lactose-based preparations should be avoided. Lactase deficiency has an incidence of about 12.5% in northern and western Europeans, and of about 80% in American Indians, Asians, blacks and Mediterraneans. Sucrose intolerance is not unknown either, in which case pilules and fine granules should not be used. However, with regard to those patients suffering from either *diabetes* or *clinical hypoglycaemia*, the quantity of sugar in a single dose is insufficient to cause any problems. The presence of even small doses of alcohol in pilules or tablets is sufficient to prohibit their use, and that of liquid alcohol potencies themselves, in the treatment of patients receiving *Antabuse* therapy for alcoholism.

Rules for the administration & storage of remedies

(1) All potentised remedies should be stored away from sunlight and perfumed substances, in tightly stoppered vials (preferably made of

amber glass). In glass, the shelf-life of correctly stored sugar-based remedies is probably no more than five years, and I would recommend discarding them after two, and obtaining new stock. In plastic vials, the same preparations should be discarded after one year. Liquid potencies, however, stored in glass, have an almost indefinite shelf-life, provided that a single succussion is applied to them about once per month. Never let the remedies be stored in any cabinet that smells of oil of cloves, nor let them be exposed to any form of intense *magnetism*. It is also a good idea to keep solid preparations away from intense sources of heat, in that dehydration may inactivate them.

(2) Solid remedies should never be directly handled. A pilule or whatever should be jiggled from the vial into its lid or a teaspoon, and then given directly into the mouth. Drops should be applied straight on the tongue with a glass pipette held at some distance. Solid remedies should be sucked, or crunched between the teeth and the fragments sucked. The full action of the remedy may not be displayed if it is immediately swallowed.

(3) Neither food nor drink should be taken for 10 minutes before and after administration.

(4) Peppermints, and mint-flavoured toothpastes may interfere with the action of the remedy, but provided that the 10 minute rule (as given above) is observed, they are unlikely to exert any significant effect.

(5) Unconscious and semiconscious patients, and small children should only be given liquid potencies, *finely crushed* pilules (or tablets) or fine granules.

(6) Dose repetition is determined by the nature and potency of the remedy, and the nature of the condition being treated. Severe acute conditions (e.g. collapse) generally require more frequent dose repetition.

(7) *Coffee*, even when decaffeinated, may be strongly antidotal to the action of many remedies, so is best avoided during treatment. Alcohol and tea in moderation are harmless. Hot spices, such as chili and ginger, seem to exert no inhibiting effect, provided that the 10 minute rule is observed.

What are the Bach Flower Remedies?

These are akin to homoeopathic remedies, but are prepared in a different manner. The supplied stock solution may be given directly into the mouth, or, as is more often the case, it is first diluted. They are useful in the treatment of psychological states. *Vervain,* however, must not be given to those suffering from *G-6-PD deficiency (favism),* where acute haemolytic anaemia may result. *Rescue Remedy* is a good all-round treatment for cases of simple shock or faint. Further details on these preparations may be obtained from a variety of books on the subject. If you are interested, you are recommended to send for the book list of the C.W. Daniel Company Ltd.

Where and how do potentised remedies act?

This matter, almost as controversial as the physicochemical basis of potentisation itself, is fully discussed in *The Infinitesimal Dose*.

The first way in which they probably act is by the stimulation of modified taste receptors within the mouth and oropharynx. This results in information being passed to the central nervous system, where it is duly processed, with the production of an appropriate set of physiological and biochemical responses. This route accounts for the extremely rapid action of some remedies. Arnica, for example, may remove the pain from a crushed finger in seconds. It also is associated, in some cases, with widespread or *constitutional* responses.

Either via the oral or pharyngeal mucosa, or via the stomach lining, the remedy is absorbed into the circulatory system, where further replication of imprinted molecules of water occurs. These then pass to the tissues where they act in two possible ways. Firstly, by occupation of the pharmacological receptor sites which would normally attract molecules of the crude drug of origin (original substance). Secondly, by the modification of hydration interactions with biological macromolecules, such as proteins and nucleic acids; that is to say by altering the properties of the aqueous environment of these biopolymers. Imprinted water molecules also pass into the breast milk, which may serve as a useful route for dosing babies.

The fate of these imprinted molecules is their energetic demotion at their various sites of action.

Proving & aggravation during treatment

These terms are related. They apply to the situation where the remedy *produces* the subjective or objective symptoms which it normally *removes*. For example, a patient taking the remedy Natrum muriaticum for coldsores may experience an increase in lesion pain, severe headache and intense thirst; all those symptoms being usually removed by that remedy. This often results from too high a potency being used (e.g. 200c), too frequent dose repetition (such as one dose per hour), or extreme subject sensitivity. In such cases, the current remedy should be discontinued. Technically, we should refer to an exaggeration of former symptoms (those related to the cold-sore) as an *aggravation*, and the new symptoms developed by the remedy as a *proving*.

How are remedies selected?

As noted previously, remedies may have a generalised or *constitutional* effect, or a more restricted action upon particular pathologies or bio-chemical dysfunctions. The latter is termed their *pathological action*; indeed, it is with this aspect of therapy that the dental surgeon is most concerned in routine practice.

In this respect, the use of a *therapeutic index* is most appropriate. This is an alphabetical index of diseases classified in the orthodox manner; following which a number of different homoeopathic treatments are given for each diagnostic entity. Most of the currently available indices are singularly useless for dental purposes. However, my former work *The Dental Prescriber*, and, more particularly, the second (encyclopaedic) section of the current book, should be found significantly more helpful.

Fortunately, in dental surgery, quite a few remedies can be prescribed upon the basis of the conventional diagnostic category alone; such as Arnica for the prevention and treatment of bruising, and Hepar sulph. for the treatment of subacute and chronic dental abscess. However, in a large number of cases, in order to prescribe satisfactorily, the objective and subjective symptoms individually manifest by the patient must also be taken into consideration. Although Chamomilla is almost routinely prescribed for teething, it may fail in cases with excessive salivation, where Mercurius solubilis is better indicated. Even the character of a pain may be of some relevance: throbbing, stabbing, burning, crushing, and so on. The *laterality* of the symptoms may also determine the selection of the remedy; Sanguinaria being more commonly indicated in right-sided migrainous neuralgia (facial migraine) and Spigelia in that involving the left side of the face. *Concomitant symptoms*, remote from the area of pathology, such as the occurrence of extreme restlessness with cold-sores, may suggest one remedy rather than another (e.g. Rhus toxico-dendron, rather than Natrum muriaticum). A good therapeutic index can simplify matters for the dental practitioner by placing the remedies in order of their overall or 'statistical' efficacy, whilst still defining their specific symptomatic indications, where these are well-established, for the more advanced 'student' of homoeopathy. Things or circumstances which make a complaint or a person better or worse (or feel that way) are termed *modalities*. In this respect, homoeopathists have borrowed the symbols < and > from mathematics, meaning 'less than' and 'greater than' respectively. In homoeopathy, however, they are taken to mean 'worse' or 'worse for' (<, lessening of health) and 'better' or 'better for' (>, increase in health). Hence, 'toothache > cold water in mouth' means that cold rinses improve the toothache.

Modalities may be classified as: *thermal* (< or > heat or cold); *climatic* (< or > rain, storms, wind, snow, humidity, change in the weather, etc.); *thermoclimatic* (e.g. < humid heat, cold winds); *periodic* or *time* (e.g. < after midnight, between 4 and 8 pm, monthly, annually, in summer); *kinetic* and *positional* (< or > movement, staying still, descent, lying on left side, etc.); *nervous* (e.g. < mental exertion, sunlight, strong odours, touch). Remember that modalities can apply to the person in general as well as to any presenting complaint. Sometimes they appear paradoxical; for example, generally < cold, but headache > cold, suggests Arsenicum album.

Constitutional aspects of pathological prescribing

Experienced prescribers often utilise an assessment of the general or *constitutional* aspects of the patient to assist them in the prescription of an appropriate remedy. For example, Natrum muriaticum is better suited to a *hot* individual (feels generally < heat) than a *chilly* one (feels generally > heat). Sepia, however, is the opposite. Therefore, in the treatment of cold-sores, where either remedy may be indicated on other grounds, 'feels generally < heat' tends to indicate Natrum mur. rather than Sepia. This is a simple example of the concept of *susceptible typology*; which essentially means that a certain type of person is sensitive to the actions of a particular remedy (or group of remedies).

Extending this concept, does this mean that Nat. mur. (as it is often so abbreviated) will have no effect on the cold-sores of a chilly person? This might be so; but, more likely, it will exert some effect, but less than it would in a hot type. The general constitution of the patient (which includes such parameters as thermal sensitivity, bodily conformation, colouring, pathological predispositions and personality) thus determines, in part, the efficacy of the pathological remedy. Hepar sulph., which almost routinely alleviates subacute or chronic dental abscesses in the majority, is actually most efficacious (swiftest in action) in those individuals who are flabby, chilly, hypersensitive to pain, and easily angered. In other words, this is the *susceptible typology* for Hepar sulph., and the individual in whom it is manifest is said to be a 'Hepar sulph. type'. The constitution is named after the remedy to which it most significantly corresponds. Similarly, we may talk of 'Phosphorus', 'Pulsatilla', 'Sulphur', 'Calcarea fluorica', 'Natrum muriaticum', and many other 'types'.

The 'pathological simillimum'

The 'pathological simillimum' is the remedy best indicated in terms of the individual symptomatology of the patient with regard to the presenting complaint (sometimes with some partial consideration of the general or constitutional aspects of the case). It is not, in view of what has been said, the *only* remedy that will act on the pathology. There is thus a certain lea-way in homoeopathic prescribing, where a remedy that is only partially indicated may still exert a certain beneficial effect. Hence, even when the most theoretically ideal remedy (the simillimum) is unavailable, a secondary remedy may often be selected, to great effect.

It should be emphasised that, whereas homoeopathists place great emphasis on individual symptomatology, the main action of the chosen pathological simillimum is upon the pathology itself. There is, however, some limited evidence (viz. its speed of action) that Arnica has some initial but limited analgesic effect in cases of bruising or crushing.

Constitutional prescribing

Constitutional prescribing implies prescription based mainly upon the general aspects of the patient (see above), rather than those related to the presenting complaint. This aspect of prescribing is more relevant to the treatment of *chronic* disease, where it is, to some degree, functionally reversible by medicinal means (such as rheumatoid arthritis, eczema, phobic disorder and predisposition to cyst formation). This usually requires much time with the patient, competent use of what is termed a *repertory* (see after), and is less suited to the ordinary dental practice. It often requires a large number of consultations and assessments (at monthly intervals or less) in order to achieve satisfactory results. Here, the *simillimum* with regard to the general or constitutional aspects of the patient, in some cases, may be difficult to assess with ease, and the 'cure' is often achieved by a sequence of different 'simillima' over the course of many months. Constitutional prescribing is particularly indicated in the treatment of chronic periodontal disease.

The matter of constitutional analysis in dental practice may, nevertheless, be simplified to a degree, with some beneficial outcome. This brings us back to the concept of *susceptible typology*, described previously. By means of a few simple parameters with regard to each case, it is possible to infer what the constitutional simillimum is likely to be. An ideal 'Pulsatilla type', for example, is placid, tearful, sensitive, initially shy, plump, fair, *thirstless*, and hot. An ideal 'Calcarea fluorica' patient exhibits weak enamel, dental overcrowding, a large angle of full extension at the elbow (greater than 180°), scoliosis of the spine, repeated sprains, lack of discipline and concentration at school (shows-off), and is < changes in climate and humidity. It is simply a matter of getting to grips with a variety of common susceptible typologies, by studying books of materia medica (Part Two of this book also gives you the more important aspects of susceptible typology of a number of common constitutional remedies). The appraisal of the patient actually begins the moment he or she enters your surgery, when you will observe such matters as general build, gait, colouring, tidiness, cleanliness, bodily odour, confidence, hostility, and so on.

Although it might seem somewhat illogical to relegate the presenting complaint to a position of secondary importance, and to favour those aspects of the patient which appear to be unrelated to it, this is not the case. Viewing a particular disease as an unhealthy tree, and the basic physiology as the soil in which it grows, it follows that we may either spray the leaves of that tree directly (pathological prescribing), or treat it by modifying the soil (constitutional prescribing). Modifying the general physiology often produces more profound and lasting cures in chronic disease than is achievable with pathological prescribing alone. Ideally, a constitutional remedy should also cover the presenting complaint and its individualised symptoms. This, however, may be difficult to achieve with a single remedy. Hence, many chronic diseases are treated with some combination or alternation of both constitutional and pathological remedies.

Where a chronic disease is incurable, due to severe and irreversible anatomical change (e.g. gross osteoarthrosis or periodontitis), or where the physiology is greatly weakened by malnutrition, chronic ill-health or age, it is often better to palliate the case with pathological remedies than to offer a constitutional prescription. In the case of severe anatomical change, little good will be achieved by a constitutional prescription. In the case of a weakened physiology, much strain will be placed upon it by such prescribing, which may, in itself, produce a further deterioration of the patient, with, in some cases, the necessity to supply an antidote. This deterioration is caused by the deployment of energy (to the treatment of a disease), the source of which is an already depleted energy pool. Always take professional advice in the treatment of such cases.

The use of the repertory

A *repertory* is quite different from a therapeutic index (see above). Although it may have a limited number of entries concerning conventional diagnostic categories, these do not comprise its main substance; not is its purpose to act as a mere substitute. The bulk of the repertory is concerned with individual objective and subjective symptoms (such as pain in the face), qualifications of those symptoms (including character, modalities and laterality), and general aspects of the patient (such as thermal sensitivity, desires, aversions, food likes and dislikes, pathological predispositions, bodily conformation, colouring, emotional status, and so on). These are classified under various headings and sub-headings termed *rubrics*. Under each rubric, a number of remedies is listed, using a variety of type faces to denote grades of importance. The idea is to select a remedy that appears to be dominantly expressed throughout a large proportion of the selected rubrics. In fact, special numerical scoring methods are taught for this purpose. In *Murphy's Homoeopathic Medical Repertory*, which is one of the most up-to-date and conveniently arranged alphabetically, remedies in **BOLD CAPITALS** score 3 points, those in ***bold italics*** score 2 points, and those in plain type score 1. Those remedies which score higher totals, when all the relevant rubrics are assessed, may be considered as significant contenders for the role of simillimum (the final judgment being made by clinical experience or by consultation of the materia medica). Whilst this technique may be applied to both pathological and constitutional prescribing, the principal application of the repertory is with regard to the latter. Here, the general aspects of the patient are more usefully *repertorised* than those of the presenting complaint (although some limited consideration of these may be relevant). In *Murphy's*, for example, we would primarily consult the chapters (or principal rubrics) headed Generals, Mind and Food (aggravations and ameliorations from, appetite, thirst, desires and aversions).

Nevertheless, the repertory still has some distinct functions in pathological prescribing. The successful use of the therapeutic index depends on the ability to make a correct orthodox diagnosis (for, it is upon such that it is based). However, no such limitation is placed upon *repertorisation*. Many cases, as exemplified by those of facial pain, are difficult to classify in conventional terms. They may be manifestations of migrainous neuralgia (facial migraine), chronic or intermittent sinusitis, chronic pulpitis, various TMJ syndromes, or mixtures of these. In a therapeutic index, we might, having made our conventional judgement, look up '***Neuralgia, migrainous***'; then choose whichever of the listed remedies

seems most appropriate under that heading. In contrast, when using a
repertory, we would refer to the individual subjective and objective *symptoms*; a method which has the advantage of being independent of the
constraints of orthodox diagnosis, which itself may be incorrect. In consulting the repertory, we must look up all the rubrics that pertain to the
case, usually starting with the location of the pain; in this case, the face,
teeth or jaws; following which, we must find those 'sub-rubrics' which
correspond to the particular character of the pain (throbbing, burning,
lancinating, etc.), those which refer to the modalities (e.g. < cold), and
those which refer to associated symptoms (such as one-sided redness of
the face). We might even look at a few relevant generals, such as thermal sensitivity and thirst, in order to complete our analysis. In this way,
the pathological simillimum may be more surely found than by scavenging through a therapeutic index. There is also, of course, the individual case where, despite a clear-cut and accurate orthodox diagnosis,
the therapeutic index fails to supply an effective remedy. Again, repertorisation is the sensible alternative.

The standard original work, of great popularity, is *Kent's Repertory* (the
structure and usage of which is explained in detail in *Bidwell's Use of the
Repertory*). However, this is actively being replaced by many contemporary books, such as that mentioned above by Murphy, which are, quite
frankly, easier to use, and which incorporate many details lacking in
Kent. For dental surgeons (and many others), *Phatak's Concise Repertory*
is probably the most suitable with which to start. Many have discovered
the apparent virtue of the computer, and have forsaken their books in
favour of it and its homoeopathic software. To date, however, it would
seem that a competent and experienced homoeopathist, armed only
with the occasional reference to a repertory, can achieve more than a
mechanician with two computers strapped to his or her side. Ultimately,
the repertory or the computer programme can only indicate what the
simillimum might be. Consultation of works of *materia medica* is necessary to confirm true clinical indications in detail; except where the
experience of the practitioner will determine the same.

The materia medica

There are numerous works on *materia medica*, where the remedies are
listed alphabetically and their properties delineated under various headings: pathological indications, susceptible typology, mind, head, eyes,
ears, nose, face, mouth, stomach, abdomen, stool, urine, male, female,
respiratory, heart, back, extremities, sleep, fever, skin, modalities,

relationship and comparison with other remedies, and dosage. Those to be recommended are *Boericke, Boger's Synoptic Key,* and *Vermeulen's Synoptic Materia Medica.* For those who wish to go into great depth, they need go no further than *Clarke's Dictionary of Materia Medica.*

Treated as a whole, the homoeopathic materia medica has many objective and subjective symptoms, the clinical significance of which has never or seldom been verified. These are symptoms which have been caused by a drug or potentised remedy (by proving), but, although the implication is that they might also be cured by the relevant remedy, this has not been satisfactorily confirmed. Good works of materia medica, however, emphasise which diseases or symptoms have been repeatedly cured by a particular remedy, so that we may be more certain in our choice (indeed, there are some entries where only the curative aspect of the remedy has been observed, and not the pathogenetic).

In homoeopathic prescribing, particularly at the constitutional level, much emphasis is often placed on the so-called *mentals*; so much so, that the mentals are separated from the *generals.* The term 'mentals' refers to the detailed psychological status of the individual (such as weepiness, loneliness, friendliness, etc.), which is often taken as a prime indication of the 'constitutional simillimum' (when an acute anxiety state in relation to dentistry is treated as an entity in itself, this is a form of pathological, rather than constitutional, prescribing).

Many of us feel, however, that the ideal selected constitutional remedy should not only cover the mental and general aspects of the case, but also those of the presenting complaint or pathology (and, preferably, with regard also to its individual symptomatic manifestation). Therefore, where two remedies would seem to be contesting on the basis of the mental and general analysis, that which more frequently treats the particular pathology should be selected in preference. In contrast to the generals, details concerning a particular pathology or disease (the presenting complaint), and its individualised objective and symptomatic picture, are termed the *particulars.*

How do we summarise the differences in use of the therapeutic index, repertory and materia medica?

In analysing any case, the initial approach is quite different with regard to the three categories of reference work:

(1) With the *therapeutic index,* we begin by selecting a category of conventional disease.

(2) With the *repertory*, we usually begin by selecting a number of general and mental characteristics, or objective and subjective symptoms.

(3) With the *materia medica*, we begin by selecting particular remedies for consideration, based upon personal clinical experience, upon the suggestions of a therapeutic index, or upon the results of repertorisation. The materia medica is thus the ultimate source of information.

What are leading symptoms?

A leading symptom is one that leads to the consideration of a limited number of remedies above all others; although often one of these is most commonly indicated, e.g. *excessive salivation and halitosis* with toothache – Mercurius sol. A leading symptom may, in fact, be a quality or modality, e.g. *throbbing* pain – Belladonna; toothache > *for cold water in the mouth* – Chamomilla (Coffea cruda also). These are leading symptoms in pathological prescribing, but the concept may be also applied to constitutional remedy selection, e.g. irritability < *especially to her nearest and dearest* – Sepia. Leading symptoms are also called *keynotes*.

However, when all is said done, a remedy might be indicated for consideration by a leading symptom, but can only be selected as appropriate if it matches the case in other respects. Irritability towards one's husband, in itself, is not a sufficient basis for the prescription of Sepia; but, where this occurs in an overworked female with bearing-down feelings in the lower abdomen, then it becomes strongly indicated. Some talk of the 'three-legged stool', implying that much good prescribing can be achieved by finding three leading symptoms which match a particular remedy. Indeed, in the hands of the expert prescriber, it is a valid technique. For those who are interested in pursuing this approach, *Nash's Leaders* is to be recommended for further reading.

Strange, rare or *peculiar* symptoms are a particular subgroup of leading symptoms, which have an enigmatic and inscrutable nature, and which lead similarly to the consideration of particular remedies (e.g. burning sensation > *heat* – Arsenicum album; urgency to urinate < *putting hands in cold water* – Kreasotum).

What is a polychrest?

A *polychrest* is a remedy of wide therapeutic applications, such as Sulphur, Arsenicum album and Calcarea carbonica. Such remedies are important in the correction of the constitution in general, and also manifest important corrective effects on a variety of pathologies.

In which potencies should we initially prescribe & with what frequency of repetition?

For newcomers to homoeopathy, it is best to restrict themselves to the prescription of either 6c or 30c, to follow the directives of the second (encyclopaedic) section of this book concerning the initial frequency of dose repetition, to withdraw the remedy if aggravation or proving occurs, and always (unless directed otherwise therein) *to discontinue treatment when significant improvement has occurred* (otherwise, aggravation or proving may result). If the case then relapses, return subsequently to the same remedy, using the same potency and repetition as before. When this fails to act satisfactorily, then an increase in the frequency of dosage or numerical potency may be indicated. If such measures fail, or consistently cause aggravation or proving, then a new remedy must be selected.

In professional prescribing for *acute* dental conditions the normal range of potencies used is actually 6–200c. The greater the *vitality* of the patient or the *severity* of the disorder, the better the indication for higher potencies. In *emotional states*, such as acute dental anxiety, higher potencies also produce a more profound and rapid effect. Additionally, it should be noted that some remedies simply act better in higher potency than lower, and vice versa. Nevertheless, despite these points, much good work can be done within the range 6–30c.

In *pathological* prescribing for *chronic* disease, it is generally advisable to restrict yourself to the use of remedies in the range 6–30c. Remedies so selected are usually given relatively frequently (often 1–3 times daily). *Constitutional* prescribing for *chronic* disease is, however, another matter. The selection of the correct remedy and dosage requires considerable experience and practice. Sometimes high or very high potencies (1M upwards) are required infrequently, or low potencies are given on a regular and frequent basis. Moreover, styles of prescribing differ considerably between different practitioners. Generally, low potency constitutional prescribing is safer for the newcomer, but it is still unwise for those who have not been properly taught.

Should a single potentised remedy be given at one time, rather than a combination?

For beginners, the answer is in the affirmative. As you develop experience, however, you may choose to give certain remedies in combination or alternation (one followed by the other in regular sequence), in order to speed the 'cure'.

In this regard, you must be aware that remedies have certain inter-relationships in terms of effect. They may be *complementary, antidotal* or *inimical.* A complementary remedy either acts synergistically with another remedy, or completes the rectification of physiology commenced by another. An antidotal remedy opposes the action of another. An inimical remedy acts with another to produce some undesirable effect (e.g. Mercurius and Silicea, given together or in alternation, may produce severe eczema). *Gibson Miller's Relationship of Remedies* is a useful and cheap reference booklet in this respect.

In professional work, constitutional and pathological remedies are often combined or alternated, in order to achieve a faster and more profound effect.

Mouthwashes (or topically applied mother tinctures) and orally administered potentised remedies may be used synergistically in therapy, provided that the mouthwash (or tincture) is not applied within 10 minutes of taking the potentised remedy.

What is Hering's Law?

Hering was one of Hahnemann's most important pupils. *Hering's Law* gives us the means of assessing the correct progression of curative (constitutional) treatment of a *chronic disease*:

'Cure occurs from above downwards, from within outwards, and in reverse chronological order.'

Put simply, this means that the cure is proceeding successfully when the upper body symptoms clear before the lower, when more important organs (e.g. the lungs) improve before those of lesser vital importance (e.g. the skin), and when old symptoms return briefly, the most recent being first manifest. Although not all these points may be observed in any particular case, the occurrence of inverse responses is regarded as an indication of incorrect therapy. Hence, where the symptoms clear from below upwards, or from the skin before the lungs, or in chronological order (the order in which they developed), then the treatment is unsatisfactory and not curative.

One thing that is not uncommon, in the successful treatment of a chronic disease, is the occurrence of a transient skin rash, even in a patient who has no history of skin disorder. This is termed *externalisation*, and is usually regarded as a strong indication that the treatment is progressing satisfactorily.

What is a miasm?

The term *miasm* is applied to various diagnostic entities in homoeopathy:

(1) A familial trait (such as thyroid disease or asthma).

(2) An inherited non-infective disease trait developed in an individual as a result of infection in the parent, which may then become a familial trait (e.g. where a parent has had TB in the past, the children subsequently born may suffer from asthma or recurrent bronchitis, and their children similarly).

(3) The prolonged aftermath of an infection or immunisation (such as ME following a viral infection, or ill-health following measles or measles immunisation).

(4) The prolonged aftermath of a drug or chemical (e.g. 'never well since an antibiotic').

Hahnemann's original miasmata (miasms) were *psora, syphilis* and *sycosis* (not *Psychosis*!). Now we have many more, including ME and the so-called *tuberculous miasm* (which covers allergy and many cases of asthma). For further details of this complex subject, you should initially consult *Jouanny's Essentials of Homoeopathic Materia Medica*. Miasmatic disease often requires the *infrequent* use of special remedies, in addition to any indicated routine constitutional treatment (such as Bacillinum for the tuberculous miasm, which may be associated with a predisposition to dental caries). Indeed, from the practical point of view, it is best to regard antimiasmatic therapy as a special area of constitutional prescribing, since it is more concerned with the 'soil' in which the disease grows.

Prescription by causation

Sometimes a remedy can be prescribed on the basis of the event, circumstances or disease which seemed to precipitate the presenting complaint or constitutional upset, even though this may have occurred many years previously. Frequently, the same remedy may be given as would have possibly been chosen for the precipitating disturbance itself. For example: epilepsy following *concussion* – Natrum sulphuricum (a principal remedy for concussion); not well since *physical trauma* – Arnica (a remedy for physical trauma); not well since *BCG immunisation* (in other words, a type of acquired tuberculous miasm) – BCG nosode; inflammatory arthritis associated with *silent periapical abscess* – Hepar sulph. (the principal remedy for chronic dental abscess).

Do drugs & remedies mix?

In general, there is no need, as far as dental matters are concerned, to interfere with any existing drug regimes prescribed by the patient's own doctor; unless, of course, they are totally without clinical effect; in which case, common sense dictates their abandonment. Potentised remedies often work extremely well, even though the patient is taking drugs (and even in the face of steroid treatment). The worst thing that can happen is that the drug will weaken the action of the remedy (which often happens when an antibiotic and a remedy are given together). Remedies seldom interfere with the action of prescribed drugs, and rarely appear to react with them to produce inimical reactions.

The importance of supplements (such as vitamins and minerals) in oral nutrition is not to be forgotten. These may be given in isolation, or alongside potentised remedies, in order to achieve maximal therapeutic effect. Those most relevant are also described in Part Two of this book.

Where do I begin?

Start with simple prescriptions, such as Arnica for the prevention of surgical haemorrhage or Hepar sulph. for subacute dental abscess. Try giving remedies for allaying anxiety, and prescribe healing mouthwashes. See what you think of *Propolis* as a disinfectant in root canal therapy. Restrict yourself initially to a pathological prescribing. With this alone you will achieve a great deal, much to your own satisfaction, and, more particularly, to that of the patient. Leave constitutional prescribing until later, when you have been taught to do it properly and you have gained sufficient experience. Otherwise, always remember that the homoeopathic physician, should he or she be well-versed in dental matters (as a number are), is there to help you.

One fine way of getting to grips with homoeopathy is to use it in your own domestic situation for common ailments, both at home and on vacation. For these general purposes, you might consult one of my previous books, *The World Travellers' Manual of Homoeopathy*. This will also give you further insight into the world-wide applications of this style of 21st Century medicine, extraordinarily conceived around 1790.

PART TWO

An Encyclopaedia of Dental Homoeopathy & Clinical Nutrition

Notes on the use of Part Two

This is not merely an encyclopaedia of homoeopathic orofacial medicine and its application to oral surgery. It is also a system of self-tuition in dental homoeopathy and nutrition, which will usefully complement the content of various courses that are available, including those of the BHDA, the British Homoeopathic Dental Association (in conjunction with the Royal London Homoeopathic Hospital).

Within its substance, each detailed topic contains a number of words or phrases emphasised in *italics*, these referring to other related headings (or rubrics). You may, therefore, start with virtually any topic in the encyclopaedia, and will be automatically led to other material. For example, **Abrasion, soft tissue** leads you to *Calendula,* and **Calendula** leads you to *fracture* and *Hypericum.* By constant cross-reference, at your own pace and in any direction you wish, you will gain an effective knowledge of basic homoeopathic dental therapeutics.

The encyclopaedia contains many entries concerning materia medica and nutritional substances referred to in therapy. These will provide you with a sound grounding in their properties, so that, at least initially, there will be no need to use this encyclopaedia along with any standard work on materia medica or nutritional supplementation. Consultation of such works, however, will become necessary at a later date, when your head has been turned and your enthusiasm fired. Major constitutional remedies are marked with an asterisk, and you should pay some attention to their susceptible typologies.

Some topics are discussed solely for the purpose of aiding differential diagnosis or providing words of caution. It is extremely unlikely these days that an early case of syphilis will be sent for homoeopathic rather than orthodox treatment. However, its relevance in the encyclopaedia is to bring its existence and nature to your attention; for, one day you may meet such a risky case, and confuse a chancre with a carcinoma or a cold-sore.

The competent practitioner must know when to treat, when to investigate, when to refer and when to collaborate.

You will note that dosages with regard to prescriptions strongly based upon the presenting complaint (so-called pathological prescriptions) are generally given in some detail; whereas those relating to constitutional prescribing are omitted (as are certain aspects of antimiasmatic prescribing). Only guidance on the selection of the constitutional simillimum is given. This is for two reasons. Firstly, constitutional prescribing requires proper tuition and experience. Secondly, styles of dosage with respect to constitutional treatment vary considerably between practitioners. Some use repeated doses of low potencies, whilst other use infrequent doses of high potencies. Others use either, according to the situation or experience, and some remedies, especially certain major nosodes (such as Bacillinum), always require infrequent repetition tailored individually to the case.

Nevertheless, since selection of the correct pathological simillimum in many instances requires some partial appraisal of the constitution, the susceptible typologies relevant to many remedies are briefly outlined. Such a knowledge of the rudiments of typology also assists the dental practitioner in communication with the professional homoeopathist. Collaboration is difficult between two people who do not speak the same language; especially one as 'strange' as that of homoeopathy, where a person may be described, for example, as a 'Phosphorus' or 'Pulsatilla' type.

It should be mentioned that those who wish to take the examinations in dental homoeopathy set by the BHDA in conjunction with the Faculty of Homoeopathy of London will find this a useful source of information. Additionally, homoeopathic practitioners themselves should find the content of considerable value in the treatment of orofacial conditions, since this subject is so neglected and poorly analysed in most of the usual homoeopathic works with which they are familiar. Neither should the homoeopathically inclined GP be disappointed in the range of topics covered.

A

Abrasion, soft tissue

These commonly occur to the lips, the corners of the mouth and the buccal mucosa, as a result of manipulation or instrumentation. Since *Calendula* is a potent promoter of the healing of damaged oral mucosa and skin, Calendula Ointment or Cream (5%) should be applied both before and after any dental procedure to the appropriate areas (some suffer from *allergy* to lanolin or chemical preservative agents, and the base must be lanolin-free or chemical preservative-free accordingly). Potentised *Arnica*, given before and after the procedure, helps to minimise bruising of the tissues.

Abscess, dental

The homoeopathic treatments of periapical and parodontal abscesses are essentially similar. Where the patient presents with significant facial swelling, *Myristica* 30 should be given immediately, followed by a further dose after about thirty minutes, and a subsequent dose one hour later. This will generally reduce the swelling and discomfort, and incision may be avoided. Thereafter, *Hepar sulph.* 6 should be given three times daily, until such time as the tooth may be root-filled or extracted, or the peridontium attended to, whichever is appropriate. Hepar sulph. given in the potency of 6c is the most successful treatment for the sub-acute and chronic dental abscess. Higher potencies, such as 30c, should not be given, since they tend to discourage proper drainage (the retention of pus prolongs the pain or discomfort, and may produce systemic disturbances). Such a prescription may indeed be pursued for many months. Where facial swelling is not a dominant feature, this remedy may be given from the outset.

Occasionally, however, other remedies will be required. *Belladonna* 30–200 every hour or two, for cases with severe *throbbing* pain. *Mercurius solubilis* 30 three times daily, for cases with gross halitosis and excessive salivation. Where the patient is feverish, give *Pyrogen* 30 three times daily, in addition to any of the selected remedies.

Hot *Calendula* or salt *mouthwashes* should also be suggested, given two or three times daily, or even more frequently in acute cases.

See also *Actinomycosis, cervicofacial; Cellulitis, acute; Endodontics; Focal sepsis; Pericoronitis; Trismus.*

***Abscess, incisional** – see* **Incisional abscess**

Aconite (Aconitum napellus)

Homoeopathic monkshood (common in Europe). Attenuations are prepared from the mother tincture of the whole plant, which is intensely poisonous. The most important remedy in acute *anxiety* states related to dentistry, especially indicated where there is great fear or dread. Also useful for the control of sudden increases in *blood pressure* in hypertensive patients as a result of dental anxiety, and attacks of *angina pectoris* from the same. In some individuals, it is capable of aborting *colds and influenza*, if given at the outset, and it can be helpful in the treatment of *Bell's palsy* and *pulpitis*. It is sometimes used constitutionally in very fearful individuals who exhibit *xerostomia*.

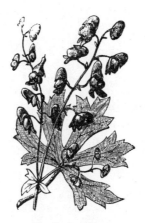

Fig. 1. Aconite

***Acquired immune deficiency syndrome** – see* **AIDS**

Acromegaly

This hormonal disorder, due to the hypersecretion of growth hormone by the pituitary gland, produces mandibular prognathism, malocclusion, spacing of the teeth, enlargement of the lips and tongue and *sialosis*. Some success in halting the progression of this disease has resulted from the long-term administration of remedies prepared from the pituitary gland itself (such as Pitressin 12), given in combination with *Calcarea carbonica*.

Actinomycosis, cervicofacial

Actinomycosis should be suspected where an abscess-like swelling appears in the region of the jaws, which, despite apparently appropriate surgical or medicinal intervention (e.g. incision, extraction, antibiotics), either remains the same or worsens after a further ten days. There may be a history of extraction or fracture in the area about 5 weeks previously. An initial induration of the tissues gives way to frank abscess formation, with the discharge of pus, containing characteristic bright yellow or grey 'sulphur granules', through multiple sinuses. Since there is the possibility of metastasis to other sites, bone erosion, and, in the case of maxillary actinomycosis, spread to the meninges, expert advice should be sought. Homoeopathy may be helpful. Initially, in the stage of induration before sinus formation, consider *Lapis albus* 6 twice daily. With sinus formation, consider *Silicea* 6–12 twice daily. Both treatments should be given in conjunction with the nosode Actinomyces israeli 30 once daily (midday).

Acupuncture

A useful adjunct to homoeopathy in the treatment of *facial pain*. Special techniques are capable of inducing anaesthesia. Recommended books for initial study are: Basics of Acupuncture by G. Stux and B. Pomeranz; The Acupuncture Treatment of Pain by L. Chaitow; and A Guide to the Location and Use of Forty-Eight Important Points by P. Vernon. Book lists are available from the East Asia Co. Ltd., 100–103 Camden High Street, London, UK.

Addison's disease

Hyposecretion of glucocorticoids and mineralocorticoids by the adrenal cortex. There is loss of weight, lethargy, hypotension, hyperpigmentation of the skin, and melanotic *pigmentation* of the oral mucosa in approximately 75% of patients (which may occur at any site). It should not be confused with racial pigmentation. Some cases are associated with *AIDS*. Replacement therapy is indicated.

Aerodontalgia

Pain in the teeth upon ascent in an aircraft. Give *Chamomilla* 30 half-hourly, or *Coffea cruda* 30 half-hourly. Cold water held in the mouth may also help.

Agranulocytosis (Granulocytopenia)
The marked diminution or absence of granular leukocytes from the bone marrow and peripheral blood. This generally occurs as a result of drug therapy having a toxic effect on the haemopoietic marrow. Potentised preparations of the offending drug may be helpful in reversing this action. It may also occur as a secondary feature of certain blood diseases, such as acute *leukaemia* and aplastic *anaemia*. Severe oral *ulcers* occur as a result of opportunistic infection. Oral *candidosis* is encouraged.

Agraphis nutans
Homeopathic bluebell. For *mouth-breathing*, where there is enlargement of adenoids and tonsils, especially when this occurs with the *eruption* of teeth. Especially indicated in chilly individuals. The **susceptible typology** is essentially similar to that of *Silicea*.

AIDS (Acquired immune deficiency syndrome)
A number of characteristic orofacial lesions are seen in AIDS cases, the recognition of which by the dental surgeon is most important. Those most frequently seen are *ANUG*, oral *candidosis, Kaposi's sarcoma, herpes simplex infection* (intraoral and perioral), *herpes zoster,* hairy *leukoplakia* and rapidly progressing *periodontitis*. More rarely, there may be *aphthous ulcers, xerostomia,* salivary gland swelling with *sialectasis, papillomavirus lesions,* non-Hodgkin's lymphoma, a brown-black *pigmentation* of the oral mucosa (possibly associated with zidovudine therapy in some), *facial nerve palsy,* trigeminal paraesthesia or anaesthesia, trigeminal *neuralgia* and *lichenoid* drug reactions. *Thrombocytopenia* also occurs. Hairy leuko-plakia is also seen in other immunocompromised patients, such as those who have undergone renal transplantation, and is thus not absolutely pathognomonic of AIDS, as was hitherto thought. Classically, it is a pain-less white lesion that affects the lateral borders of the tongue. Oral candidosis may be of the pseudomembranous, hyperplastic or erythe-matous type, and candida-related *angular cheilitis* and *median rhomboid glossitis* also occur. Homoeopathy may be helpful in the control of AIDS and its various manifestations, including the use of an AIDS nosode.

Albers-Schönberg disease – see **Osteopetrosis**

Albright's syndrome – see **Fibrous dysplasia**

Allergy, food – see **Food allergy**

Allergy, orofacial

The occurrence of oral ulceration, oedema of the lip, gingivitis or mucosal white patches may be associated infrequently with sensitivity to dental materials (such as *amalgam*), *toothpastes*, or constituents of *food* or drink. Special testing (such as the patch test) may be required to identify the allergen. Allergy may be implicated in *aphthous ulcers, burning mouth syndrome, denture sore mouth, erythema multiforme*, chronic atrophic *gingivitis* (in relation to restorations or chrome prostheses), *lichenoid reactions* and *orofacial granulomatosis*. Rarely, allergy may be related to local *anaesthesia*. *Angioedema* is a condition which simulates true allergy. Allergy to lanolin, the active constituent, or preservative in creams or ointments occasionally occurs.

See also *Bacillinum*.

Allium sativum

Homoeopathic garlic. A remedy for *sialorrhoea* after eating. **Susceptible typology:** voracious carnivores, overindulgent, dyspeptic (certain similarities to the *Nux vomica* type), tongue pale with red papillae. Ordinary garlic is taken for *candidosis*.

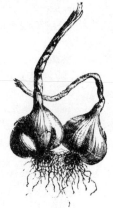

Fig. 2. Allium Sativum

Aloe vera

A botanic vulnerary. One of several species of Aloes, and not to be confused with the Aloe socatrina of homoeopathy. The fresh juice of the fleshy leaves is antifungal, and may be used to treat oral *candidosis*. A mouthwash may be prepared by adding 10ml of the juice to 250ml of water, to be used 3–4 times daily. Alternatively, it may be incorporated

(5%) in a cream. It may be mixed with *Berberis vulgaris* and *Hydrastis canadensis*. Aloe vera is also sometimes used as an application to *aphthous ulcers*.

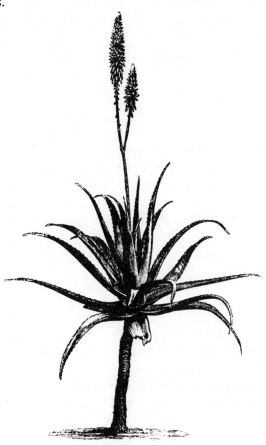

Fig. 3. Aloe vera

Amalgam, dental

This substance may be potentised to produce a remedy to oppose any *mercury toxicity* (see *Appendix 2*) consequent upon the removal of old amalgam fillings. It should not be used in a potency of less than 6c or 11x (D11). Amalgam fillings themselves may be associated locally with *lichenoid reactions* of the oral mucosa and *amalgam tattoos*. Emitted mercury vapour is associated with the development of *antibiotic* resistance by the bacterial flora of the oronasal region. Removal of amalgam is sometimes followed by unusual symptomatic pictures, presumably resulting from inhalation of mercury vapour. These may be antidoted by homoeopathic means, with prescriptions based upon the individual symptomatology which develops. The most commonly indicated remedies in this respect are *Aurum metallicum, Carbo vegetabilis, Hepar sulph.*, Kali iodatum, *Lachesis, Natrum sulphuricum, Nitricum acidum, Phytolacca, Staphysagria* and *Sulphur*. Some skill is involved in their selection, and reference to detailed repertories is sometimes required.

Amalgam tattoo

The presence of amalgam fragments within the oral mucosa may lead to a bluish patch of oral mucosa. This is initially radio-opaque, but subsequently becomes radiolucent. Amalgam also appears to be able to pass electrophoretically from filled teeth into the oral mucosa; and such tattoos are always radiolucent. These patches must be differentiated from other causes of intraoral *pigmentation*, such as *melanoma* and *Kaposi's sarcoma*. Amalgam tattoos are an unlikely source of *mercury toxicity* (see *Appendix 2*), in that this is mainly related to mercury vapour.

Ambra grisea

Homoeopathic ambergris (from the whale). Used in the treatment of some cases of *ranula*. **Susceptible typology:** extraordinarily timid children and adults, the adults being prematurely aged (*Pulsatilla* types may be timid to varying degrees, but tend to appear younger than their years; *Lycopodium* types are prematurely aged, but not outwardly timid).

Amphisbaena (Amphisbaena vermicularis)

Homoeopathic preparation of a snake-like lizard. Given for mandibular *osteomyelitis*, especially of the right side, with pain < air, < dampness, < motion, < afternoon and < evening. May be used for *toothache* with the same modalities.

Amyloidosis

The extracellular deposition of amyloid protein is one cause of macroglossia, as is *hypothyroidism* in infants. Surgery may be indicated. The homoeopathic treatment of both localised and widespread amyloidosis is complex.

Anaemia

Anaemia is not uncommonly associated with *iron, folate* or *vitamin B12* deficiency. The dental surgeon may tentatively diagnose anaemia from oral symptoms and signs. Aplastic anaemia, due to failure of haemopoiesis within the marrow, is characterised by haemorrhagic lesions of the gingivae and oral mucosa, and opportunistic oral infection.

See also *Agranulocytosis*.

Anaesthesia, general

In order to prevent chest infections in chesty patients, give *Antimonium tartaricum* 6 three times daily, for several days before and one week after the procedure (this may be used in conjunction with *Arnica*, *Hypericum* or *Pyrogen*, given for other reasons). To arouse patients after general anaesthesia, give *Opium* 100–200 (liquid potency) quarter-hourly; *Phosphorus* 30 (liquid potency) or higher is an alternative. If the patient is nauseated, give *Ipecacuanha* 30 (liquid potency) quarter-hourly.

For those interested in the more esoteric effects of nitrous oxide, they might take note of the story quoted by Bertrand Russell: 'William James describes a man who got the experience from laughing gas; whenever he was under its influence, he knew the secret of the universe, but when he came to, he had forgotten it. At last, with immense effort, he wrote down the secret before the vision had faded. When completely recovered, he rushed to see what he had written. It was "A smell of petroleum prevails throughout".'

Anaesthesia, local

The routine use of *Arnica* before and after dental procedures tends to prevent *haematoma* formation. True *allergy* to local anaesthetics is rare, and general symptoms that arise (e.g. nausea and dizziness) are more likely associated with accidental intravenous administration or *anxiety*. *Smelling salts* are sometimes invaluable in such a situation. Fischer recommends *Chamomilla* 30 for any systemic or psychic effects of local anaesthesia. Where stiffness of the jaw persists after an injection of local anaesthetic, particularly after an inferior dental nerve block, consider *Ledum* 30 three or four times daily. Occasionally, *Ruta* 30–200 three or four times daily (or initially more frequently, according to response) is better indicated, where the pain is felt in the bone as a result of scraping the periosteum, or as a result of intra-alveolar injection. An obvious haematoma is better treated with Arnica. *Apis* 30 three times daily is given for oedema at the injection site, with burning or stinging pains > cold applications. *Hypericum* 30–200 three or four times daily (or more frequently) is indicated where the nerve trunk has been damaged by the needle, and there are shooting pains. Local anaesthesia of the palate may be contributory to the development of *necrotising sialometaplasia*.

See also *Oral surgery, pain control after*.

Angina bullosa haemorrhagica (ABH)
Recurrent intraoral blood blisters. ABH is sometimes associated with steroid therapy, given systemically or by inhaler. A solitary blood-filled blister develops in seconds or minutes, usually upon the soft palate, and sometimes associated with the ingestion of food. The blister bursts spontaneously within 24 hours, leaving an *ulcerated* area which heals within 7–10 days. Usually 5–10 episodes occur over 2–3 years. *Thrombocytopenia* should be excluded by blood test. Immediate treatment includes puncturing the intact blister. Also give *Arnica* 30 three times daily for up to 10 days. *Calendula* mouthwashes should be used three times daily, in order to promote healing.

Angina, Ludwig's – *see* Cellulitis, acute

Angina pectoris
Characterised by transient retrosternal pain, radiating to the neck or left arm, this may occur as a result of acute dental *anxiety*. In addition to any regular medication used by the patient for such an emergency, remedies may be given to assist, such as *Aconite* or *Bach* Rescue Remedy. Alternatively, *Latrodectus* 30 may be given in the same manner as Aconite. Obviously, the persistence of pain, despite rest and medicinal therapy, is more suggestive of myocardial infarction, and medical advice should be urgently sought.

Angioedema
Recurrent non-allergic oedema of the tongue or lips, often precipitated by trauma. It may be associated with drug therapy (particularly anti-hypertensive agents) or it may be genetic in origin. Tongue swelling may cause difficulty in breathing. Some cases have responded to potentised *Sulphur*.

Angular cheilitis (Perlèche)
A painful fissure of the corner of the mouth, often occurring bilaterally. Infection is often present, involving candida organisms, staphylococcus aureus, or, more rarely, haemolytic streptococci. Angular cheilitis may be associated with oral *candidosis* (including that related to poor denture

hygiene), *iron* deficiency (including that related to *rheumatoid arthritis*), *vitamin B2* deficiency, *folate* deficiency, *vitamin B12* deficiency, *diabetes mellitus*, *orofacial granulomatosis*, *AIDS* and *Crohn's disease*. Angular cheilitis is occasionally confused with recurrent *herpes labialis*, erosive *lichen planus* or facial eczema. The role of severe overclosure in its aetiology is unclear.

Despite the multiplicity of causative factors, many cases clear up with vitamin B2 supplementation, 50mg once daily (adult dose), or 25mg daily for most children. You should warn your patients that their urine will become bright yellow in colour. Treatment is often necessary for several months at a time, and a discontinuation may be followed by relapse, necessitating represcription of the vitamin. The origin of the local deficiency state is unclear, and is not necessarily caused by an inadequate diet. Some form of malabsorption may be at the root of the matter. It is not generally necessary to give other B vitamins in conjunction with B2, despite the protestations of the naturopaths, since the diet will usually contain adequate amounts of these. Treatment may be accelerated by the use of an antifungal and antibacterial topical application, composed of 50g of aqueous cream in which has been mixed 5–10 drops of *tea tree oil*, applied two or three times daily (where staphylococcal infection has been confirmed, the anterior nares should be treated with the same). Should such simple treatment fail, then investigation of the underlying cause with be necessary (e.g. blood tests for iron deficiency). Appropriate fundamental treatment should then be instituted. Where candida infection has been confirmed, treatment for intraoral candidosis may be necessary.

Anorexia nervosa & bulimia nervosa
Both these conditions are of psychopathological origin. Anorexia nervosa is characterised by the avoidance of food and recurrent vomiting. Bulimia nervosa is characterised by gluttony, followed by self-induced vomiting. Both conditions may be improved by professional homoeopathic treatment, and *zinc* supplementation is certainly useful in anorexic cases. The exposure of the teeth to gastric acid produces erosion of the enamel. Bilateral parotid *sialosis* also occurs.

Anthracinum
Homoeopathic. Anthrax nosode. Used in the treatment of *anthrax*, recurrent boils and *cancrum oris*.

Anthrax

This bacterial disease may be identified sometimes by the dental surgeon where it occurs on the face. The characteristic appearance is a solitary papule with a black necrotic centre ('malignant pustule'), surrounding vesicles and oedema. It is most common in those who work with animals or animal materials: butchers, tanners, vets. A fatal septicaemia can result. Both allopathic and homoeopathic therapies are available, including the use of the nosode *Anthracinum*.

Antibiotics, ill-effects of

The use of antibiotics is largely avoidable by the judicious prescription of homoeopathic remedies. Three common complications of antibiotic therapy are thrush (oral or vaginal candidosis), diarrhoea and allergic skin rash. Thrush may be treated internally with *Borax* 30–200 three times daily (see also *candidosis, oral*). Diarrhoea may be treated with either *Crataegus* Ø 5 drops in a little water three times daily (adult dose), or *Nitricum Acidum* 30 4-hourly. The disappearance of an allergic skin rash may be hastened by giving *Thuja* 6 two or three times daily.

See also *Tongue, black hairy*.

Anti-inflammatory drugs

These are commonly employed in the treatment of musculoskeletal injuries and inflammations. They may produce *lichenoid reactions*.

Antimonium crudum

Homoeopathic preparation of native antimony sulphide. Used for loss of *taste* with a thick creamy coating on the *tongue*, and in the treatment of *impetigo*. **Susceptible typology:** irritable, dyspeptic, nails thick and hard (split longitudinally), < cold bathing and direct heat of a fire or the sun, > hot baths and applications.

Antimonium tartaricum

Homoeopathic preparation of tartar emetic. Given for loss of *taste* with a thick white coating on the *tongue*, which has red edges; especially in chesty subjects. Used also in the prevention of chest infection following general *anaesthesia*, and in the treatment of *chickenpox*.

ANUG – *see* Gingivitis, acute necrotising ulcerative

Anxiety, acute dental (Odontophobia)

Acute anxiety, apprehension and fear are not uncommon both before and during dental procedures, in both adults and children. Remedies improve the psychological status, without the drugging effect associated with conventional tranquillisers. The most important remedy to be considered is *Aconite*. The main indications for Aconite are fear, dread, panic or psychological shock. Since one or more of these is usually present in most cases of acute dental anxiety, Aconite is commonly indicated, especially where the mouth is dry. Mild cases may respond to a 30c, but higher potencies (200–1M) are often required for more severe states, particularly where a rapid action is required. Initial repetition may be quite frequent (every 15 minutes) in the dental surgery. The same remedy may be given less frequently (three or four times daily) for several days before the next visit. Some favour the use of *Bach* Rescue Remedy as an alternative to Aconite.

Occasionally, Aconite (or Rescue Remedy) is unsuccessful, and other remedies are required, given with the same frequency of repetition. *Argentum nitricum* 30–200 is indicated where the patient becomes excessively talkative as a result of anxiety, and is constantly on the move (sits down and gets up frequently, reads one magazine for a few minutes, plays with and looks at his or her watch constantly, reads another magazine). In contrast, *Gelsemium* 30–200 is indicated where the patient is uncommunicative, inactive and trembling. Diarrhoea may accompany the other symptoms of either the Gelsemium or the Argentum nitricum case. *Coffea cruda* 30–200 is suited to those who are overenthusiastic, sleepless (mind full of thoughts) and excessively sensitive to pain. As with Aconite, the prescription of these remedies for a few days before the next visit may be helpful. Occasionally, *Chamomilla* is also indicated in adult cases, as is *Ignatia*.

Fischer feels that the most commonly indicated remedies in acute dental anxiety are Aconite, Coffea, Gelsemium, Ignatia and *Arsenicum album*. A leading indication for Coffea is that the patient is very sensitive to noise of any sort, and insists that any background music is turned off; toothaches tend to be better for cold water held in the mouth. Ignatia patients are made to feel extremely ill by coffee or tobacco smoke, and their general anxiety often stems from an unpleasant psychological shock in the past (e.g. loss of a loved one, being jilted or rejected). Arsenicum album is indicated in extremely chilly and fastidious patients, who have profound anxieties about their health and may experience burning pains > heat. Any of these remedies may be given in the range of 30–200c, according to the degree of psychological disturbance, with repetition according to response.

Both *Arnica* and *Hypericum*, which are routinely given by many before and after dental procedures, are compatible with all the above remedies, and may be given concurrently.

See also *Children, fractious*.

Aphthous ulcers (Recurrent aphthous stomatitis, RAS)

These are usually classified as major (MaRAS), minor (MiRAS) and herpetiform (HU). MiRAS is the most common form (80%), and is characterised by *ulcers* no more than 5 mm in diameter, and 1–6 in number. They do not occur on the palate or in the throat. Spontaneous healing occurs within 14 days, with no residual scarring. The interval between attacks is highly variable. MaRAS is less common (10%), and is characterised by ulcers that are 1–3 cm in diameter, which may appear anywhere in the mouth or oropharynx, which may persist for one month or more, and which heal with the production of *scars*. HU is the least common type, with up to 100 small herpetiform ulcers being present at one time. These most commonly occur in the floor of the mouth and at the tip and lateral margins of the tongue. They may last from 7–14 days, and heal without scarring. RAS must be differentiated from *carcinoma* (MaRAS), simple traumatic ulcer (MiRAS), as from a sharp tooth, *herpes simplex infection* (HU) and some forms of erosive *lichen planus*.

Occasionally RAS may be brought on by *allergy* to certain foods, especially chocolate and preservatives (see also *orofacial granulomatosis*). RAS can be associated with *AIDS*, psychological stress (including acute dental *anxiety* and 'pre-exam nerves'), *iron* deficiency (including that associated with *rheumatoid arthritis*), *vitamin B1* deficiency, *vitamin B6* deficiency, *vitamin B12* deficiency, *zinc* deficiency, oral trauma (development of ulcers at traumatic sites), the menstrual cycle, *coeliac disease*, *Crohn's disease* and *ulcerative colitis*. There may be an inherited miasmatic (miasmic) predisposition in some cases. RAS may also be a manifestation of *Behçet's disease*.

Contrary to the views generally expressed in both conventional and homoeopathic literature, this unpleasant condition is not particularly difficult to treat in the majority of patients. There are two aspects to treatment: that for the immediate complaint, and that for the predisposition.

Immediate relief from pain may be obtained by dispersing 4–8 drops (or more if necessary) of *Propolis* Ø in 10 ml of warm water, and holding the solution in the mouth in contact with the lesion, for a few minutes until it has taken effect (alternatively, the undiluted Ø may be used directly, but this will sting). Some then recommend swallowing the solution, but I do not. This may be repeated several times daily. Propolis is actually a potent promoter of healing in cases of aphthous ulceration. *Myrrh* Ø, which also has its proponents, may be used in a similar way to Propolis, but should not be swallowed. An infusion of dried or fresh kitchen sage (about 1 teaspoon to 1 teacup of hot water, allowed to stand for 10 minutes) is a useful *mouthwash* where neither Propolis nor Myrrh is available; it too should not be swallowed. As far as internal treatment is concerned, which may be used in conjunction with topical therapies, *Feverfew* 30 three times daily helps many cases. This remedy may even abort the frank development of ulceration if given in the premonitory tingling phase. Other remedies require consideration, where Feverfew is ineffective. In nervous and timid patients (especially if they are very sensitive to loud noises), consider *Borax* 30 4-hourly. Where there is foul breath, copious saliva and the tongue retains the imprint of the teeth, *Mercurius Solubilis* 6–30 4-hourly is indicated. Again, where the tongue bears the imprint of the teeth, but the breath is inoffensive and the saliva is thick and tenacious, *Hydrastis* 30 4-hourly should be given. For ulcers with yellow or yellow-green bases, consider *Kali bichromicum* 30 4-hourly. Where the base of the ulcer bleeds easily and there are sticking or splinter-like pains, give *Nitricum acidum* 30 4-hourly. *Natrum muriaticum* 6–30 two or three times daily is indicated where the ulcers are brought on by baking-soda toothpaste.

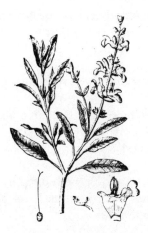

Fig. 4. Salvia officinalis (kitchen sage)

For the treatment of the predisposition, in conjunction with remedies, zinc 15–30mg daily (adult dose) should be given to all cases. Feverfew 30 twice daily, given long-term, is helpful in many. More resistant cases often require potentised *Sulphur*. However, even before considering its use, the practitioner should rule out the possibility of deficiency states (for which supplementary therapy will be required), allergic states (where exclusion will be beneficial), and any coexistent pathologies (for which special treatment will be indicated). Sulphur treatment itself is to be used cautiously, since it is prone to cause skin eruptions of various types (eczema, pimples or boils), whereupon it must be discontinued until professional advice can be obtained. A relatively safe starting prescription is Sulphur 6 twice daily for a few months. However, difficult cases may require potencies of up to 200c; but these must only be given intermittently and by those with good clinical experience. Constitutional treatment, based upon the general and mental characteristics of the patient, may be occasionally required. In hormonally-dependent cases in women, remedies with an affinity for pituitary-ovarian axis, such as *Sepia* and Natrum muriaticum, according to their proper indications, may be of service, along with *evening primrose oil*. *Bach flower remedies* may be helpful in cases which are brought on by circumstantial psychological stress or personality disorders. *Argentum nitricum* 30–200 twice daily is a major remedy in the treatment of RAS brought on by hyperactive 'pre-exam nerves'.

Fischer's technique for treating aphthous ulcers is worthy of mention. A drop of the oily contents of a *vitamin E* capsule or *Aloe vera* extract is applied occasionally to each ulcer. L-lysine (an amino acid) 1 g per meal three times daily (adult dose) is given until the ulcers have cleared. At the same time arginine (another amino acid) must be reduced. This is especially found in chocolate, peanuts, other nuts, seeds, cereal grains, gelatin, raisins and carob; and these should be excluded from the diet for a prolonged period or indefinitely. Once the ulcers have cleared, the dose of L-lysine is reduced to 500mg per meal three times daily. A maintenance dose of 500mg daily is sometimes necessary to prevent recurrence. L-lysine reduces the severity of the disorder and promotes healing. However, it may cause an increase in levels of cholesterol and triglycerides, and these should be monitored in patients on extended therapy. A similar approach has been used, to some effect in the treatment of *herpes simplex infection*.

Apis (Apis mellifica)

Homoeopathic preparation of the honey-bee. A remedy for reactive oedema and *cellulitis*, with burning and stinging pains, < heat, > cold. If fever is present, the patient is thirstless. Indicated in some cases of *neuralgia* with burning and prickling sensations, and *pulpitis* or post-local *anaesthetic* pain with the same modalities. It is especially indicated in persons of *Natrum muriaticum* **typology**.

Apprehension – see **Anxiety, acute dental**

Aranea diadema

Homoeopathic preparation of Papal-Cross spider. Given for *neuralgia*, especially right-sided. This remedy has two leading symptoms: exact periodicity (symptoms come on always at the same hour of the day), and a sensation of great swelling of the affected part. Other indications include: < cold humidity, and nocturnal *toothache*.

Argentum metallicum

Homoeopathic preparation of silver. A remedy for *laryngitis* of talkative dentists, with pain in the larynx < swallowing and talking, especially with the coughing up of thick mucus.

Argentum nitricum*

Homoeopathic preparation of silver nitrate. Useful in certain acute dental *anxiety* states and in the treatment of acute purulent *conjunctivitis*. It is also a principal remedy for 'pre-exam nerves' (with a picture of hyperactivity) and *aphthous ulcers* stemming therefrom, irrespective of the normal susceptible typology of the patient. It is sometimes indicated in the treatment of *median rhomboid glossitis*. **Susceptible typology:** thin, withered, forgetful, excited, hurried, anxious, incompetent, fear of heights, phobic (e.g. agoraphobic), hypoglycaemic (< sweets), < intellectual work, chronic pharyngitis (clears throat repeatedly), prone to stomach problems (distention, epigastric pain, ulcers).

Arnica (Arnica montana)

Homoeopathic and botanic. Leopard's bane, which grows in mountainous areas. The mother tincture is prepared from the roots or whole plant (if the flowers are infested with the Arnica fly, they are unsuitable). The mother tincture is not suitable for systemic or oral use, even when diluted. It is, however, usefully applied externally to bruises, *haematomata* and *sprains*, several times daily, provided that the skin is intact (even so, in rare instances, an allergic eczema may result). It must not be applied to broken skin, even when diluted. Systemically, it must be used in its potentised form, usually in a 30c, but may be given in any potency from 6 to 200. It is the most important remedy for the prevention and treatment of bruising and *haemorrhage*, thus indirectly promoting healing. It should be given both before and after all dental procedures where trauma to the tissues is involved. The basic dose repetition is three times daily, but, where there is much bleeding (as with *oral surgery*), it may be given as often as once ever 15 minutes. Along with Arnica, *Hypericum* is also routinely given by many, three times daily, in order to oppose nerve damage. Arnica should be given to all those who have suffered severe physical trauma (e.g. from road traffic accidents), where again it may be repeated frequently. Virtually all patients benefit from Arnica, whose only near, but less effective, rival is *Bellis perennis*. Apart from its antihaemorrhagic effect, Arnica appears to have some mild central analgesic effect in cases of physical trauma. Arnica is the remedy *par excellence* for the control of pain associated with bruised soft tissues. It may also be used internally in the treatment of acute sprains, and *angina bullosa haemorrhagica*.

See also *Dislocation, TMJ; Oral surgery, pain control after.*

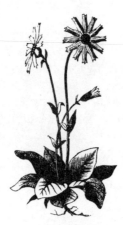

Fig. 5. Arnica

Arsenicum album*

Homoeopathic prepration of arsenic trioxide. Useful in some cases of acute dental *anxiety*, malignant *tumour, pemphigus, pemphigoid, pulpitis, halitosis, burning mouth syndrome, lichen planus,* atrophic *gingivitis, median rhomboid glossitis* and *xerostomia*. **Susceptible typology:** pale, thin, chilly (to the core), meticulous in all respects, smartly dressed, children fragile and elegant, alternating and changing mood, easily frightened, extreme anxiety about illness, very weak with all ailments, burning pains > heat, headaches < heat, < after midnight, marked thirst for small rations of water taken frequently, prone to allergies and asthma, *tongue* indented.

Arteritis, giant cell – see **Giant cell arteritis**

Arthritis, odontogenic – see **Focal sepsis**

Arthritis, rheumatoid – see **Rheumatoid arthritis**

Arum triphyllum
Homoeopathic preparation of Jack in the pulpit. A remedy for *laryngitis* in talkative dentists, where the voice is continually changeable from hoarse to clear. Also useful in disorders of the *TMJ*.

Ascorbic acid – see **Vitamin C**

Aspirin burn
Holding an Aspirin tablet against a painful tooth leads to a chemical burn of the oral mucosa. *Calendula* or Calendula and *Hypericum* mouthwashes, ointments and creams promote healing.
  See also *von Willebrand's disease*.

Atypical facial pain – see **Facial pain, atypical**

Atypical odontogenic pain – see **Facial pain, atypical**

Auriculo-temporal syndrome – see **Frey's syndrome**

Aurum metallicum
Homoeopathic gold. A remedy for *halitosis* or *gingivitis* of girls at puberty, especially if they are very gloomy or depressive. Also employed in the treatment of *Paget's disease*.

B

Bach flower remedies

An important group of liquid medicines, allied in function and use to homoeopathic remedies, and generally given in aqueous dilution. A satisfactory dose is 3–4 drops. Most are given to good effect three times daily, but Rescue Remedy, which is similar to *Aconite* in action, may be used frequently (ever 5 minutes, if necessary) in cases of *collapse*, faint, or acute dental *anxiety*. Their principal sphere of action is the psyche, but, where psychosomatic disorders are present, they will exert an indirect action upon the physiology. They are administered upon the basis of the psychological status of the patient, including their general personality. They can usually be given in conjunction with true homoeopathic remedies, and only rarely produce aggravations. It is customary to mix several together in order to cover the case more fully, but I do not recommend the use of more than three at one time. In dentistry, they are particularly helpful in some cases of migrainous *neuralgia*, *aphthous ulcers*, atypical *facial pain* and *craniomandibular dysfunction*, where the psyche is at fault. Such psychological problems may be circumstantial (e.g. bereavement) or personality-dependent (e.g. tendency to suppress emotions). The remedies, together with their principal indications, are as follows:

(1) **Agrimony**. Conceals tensions behind a brave face (conscious suppression).

(2) **Aspen**. Fears things for no logical reason.

(3) **Beech**. Intolerant, orderly and antisocial.

(4) **Centaury**. Timid, easily imposed upon, weak-willed.

(5) **Cerato**. Doubts own ability, saps the vitality of others by constantly seeking advice and confirmation.

(6) **Cherry Plum**. Fear of mind giving away and losing control of temper.

(7) **Chestnut Bud**. Failure to learn from past misjudgments.

(8) **Chicory**. Argumentative, possessive, selfish.

(9) **Clematis**. Day-dreamers.

(10) **Crab Apple**. Self-disgust.

(11) **Elm**. Essentially competent people who are overwhelmed by work or responsibility (the 'teacher's remedy').

(12) **Gentian**. Easily discouraged by minor setbacks.

(13) **Gorse**. Convinced he or she will never be cured.

(14) **Heather**. Self-concern, obsessed with ailments. Obsessive-compulsive disorders.

(15) **Holly**. Jealousy, hatred, envy (the 'cheated party remedy').

(16) **Honeysuckle**. Homesickness, unpleasant nostalgia, prolonged bereavement.

(17) **Hornbeam**. Mental fatigue, prolonged convalescence.

(18) **Impatiens**. Impatient and irritable.

(19) **Larch**. Lack of confidence but not ability.

(20) **Mimulus**. Fear of known things.

(21) **Mustard**. Deep depression without circumstantial cause.

(22) **Oak**. Solid and reliable types who soldier on through difficulties, and suffer accordingly.

(23) **Olive**. Total exhaustion of mind and body.

(24) **Pine**. Guilt.

(25) **Red Chestnut**. Anxiety about the welfare of others.

(26) **Rock Rose**. Panic, terror.

(27) **Rock Water**. Self-repression, concerned with self-perfection.

(28) **Scleranthus**. Indecisive.

(29) **Star of Bethlehem**. Shock, fright.

(30) **Sweet Chestnut**. Utter despair.

(31) **Vervain**. Overdoers of things, perfectionistic, sensitivity to injustice.

(32) **Vine**. Inflexible and domineering.

(33) **Walnut**. Ill-effects of change in circumstances or domination by another person.

(34) **Water Violet**. Aloof and proud.

(35) **White Chestnut**. A distressing or worrying event or situation prays on the mind (the 'litigation remedy').

(36) **Wild Oat**. Inability to decide one's future course in life.

(37) **Wild Rose**. Resignation to one's lot in life, too apathetic to change.

(38) **Willow**. Resentment.

(39) **Rescue Remedy** (this remedy is a mixture of Impatiens, Cherry Plum, Clematis, Rock Rose, and Star of Bethlehem). Collapse, faint, acute anxiety.

A knowledge of the Bach Flower Remedies is not required for the BHDA examination.

Bacillinum

Homoeopathic. A nosode of tuberculous lung. A remedy for the tuberculous miasm. It is sometimes indicated in cases of delayed *eruption* and *mouth-breathing.* Occasionally it is used for cases of *bruxism* in children. It may be helpful in reducing a predisposition to either dental *caries* or orofacial *allergy.* It has been used in the treatment of *sarcoidosis.* A red stripe down the centre of *tongue* may be indicative of its applicability. It is given in infrequent dosages and should only be used by the competent practitioner.

Baptisia (Baptisia tinctoria)

Homoeopathic wild indigo. A remedy for primary herpetic *gingivo-stomatitis* with fetid breath and severe prostration.

Behçet's disease (Behçet's syndrome)

This miasmatic (miasmic) disease, first recognised by Hippocrates, has a high prevalence in Japan and countries bordering the Mediterranean. It is more common in males. Characteristically, there are oral and genital *ulcers,* and ocular lesions, but other associated disorders may be present. Recurrent oral ulceration is typical, with three or more attacks occurring within one year. This takes the form of major aphthous, minor aphthous or herpetiform ulceration. Genital aphthous ulceration, with scarring, dysuria and pain on intercourse, is common. Ocular lesions occur in most cases, including anterior uveitis, posterior uveitis, conjunctival ulceration and retinal vasculitis. Scarring and blindness may result. Other disorders include: arthritis, recurrent thombophlebitis, neurological disorders and gastrointestinal disturbances.

Topical treatment, as described for *aphthous ulcers,* is useful. Homoeopathic treatment may be complex, but *Sulphur* appears to be a key remedy in therapy.

Belladonna

Homoeopathic deadly nightshade. Useful for early *abscess* and acute *cellulitis.* It is well-indicated where there is a sudden onset of swelling, accompanied by redness, intense heat (with burning sensation) and *throbbing* pain. The face is often red and congested.

In febrile states, there is a great thirst for cold water. It is sometimes given for cases of *bruxism* or bruxomania, where the muscles of the jaw are burning or throbbing, especially in ruddy-faced individuals. Also indicated in some cases of *pulpitis.* Belladonna is most effective in robust individuals.

See also *Endodontics.*

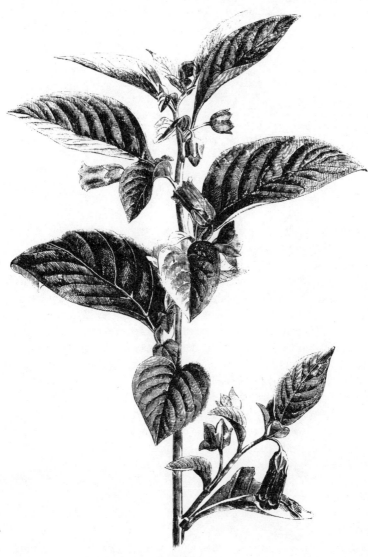

Fig. 6. Belladonna

Bellis perennis

Homoeopathic wound-wort (a common daisy). Similar in action to *Arnica*, but perhaps slightly weaker. It is also a valuable remedy for 'gardener's backache', and is generally used in a potency of 30c. Rather like

Arnica, it may be used frequently (as often as ever 15 minutes) in cases of trauma, or less frequently (say, three times daily) in cases of lumbago.

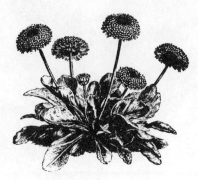

Fig. 7. Bellis perennis

Bell's palsy

In this disease of acute onset, there is a non-traumatic unilateral lower motor neurone lesion of the *facial nerve*, possibly of viral origin. Occasionally, there is some loss of taste on the affected side. It may be clinically differentiated from an upper motor neurone lesion (e.g. from a cerebrovascular haemorrhage) by asking the patient to raise the eyebrow of the affected side. Characteristically, the Bell's palsy patient is incapable of doing so, whereas this ability is generally preserved in upper motor neurone cases. Treatment should begin as soon as possible with *Aconite* 30 and *Causticum* 30 given in alternation; 2-hourly alternation in early cases (within 48 hours of onset), or 4-hourly alternation in later cases. Facial nerve paralysis of gradual onset is indicative of either intracranial or parotid *tumour*.

See also *AIDS; Lyme disease; Melkersson-Rosenthal syndrome; Ramsay-Hunt syndrome.*

Berberis vulgaris

Botanic and homoeopathic. Barberry. For dental purposes, the mother tincture, which is prepared from the root bark, is mainly of interest. It may be used in the treatment of oral *candidosis*, either as a mouthwash (30 drops Ø in 250ml of water) to be used 3–4 times daily, or in the form of a 5% cream or ointment. It may be mixed with *Aloe vera* and *Hydrastis canadensis*.

Fig. 8. Berberis vulgaris

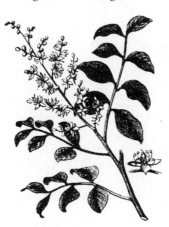

Biliary cirrhosis, primary

This chronic disease of the liver, insidious in onset and usually occurring in women aged 40–60, may be accompanied by *Sjögren's syndrome*.

Bioflavonoids

These valuable food substances act with *vitamin C* in maintaining collagen structure, and reducing and preventing inflammation, bleeding and infection in the periodontium. Mixed bioflavonoids 500mg three times daily are sometimes prescribed in cases of *gingivitis* or *periodontitis*.

Bitten cheek or tongue

Give potentised *Arnica* internally, and prescribe *Calendula* mouthwashes.
  See also *Cheek biting, recurrent.*

Blastomycosis – *see* Fungal diseases

Bleeding, surgical – *see* Haemorrhage, acute dental

Blood pressure, acute elevation of

Hypertensive patients suffering from apprehension or distress may experience a sudden elevation of blood pressure, with the development of symptoms, such as headache and *epistaxis*. They should be given *Aconite* along the lines suggested for acute dental *anxiety*, and referred to their own physicians. Hypertensive epistaxis may require additional treatment with *Ferrum phosphoricum*.

Blow to a tooth – *see* Traumatised tooth

Bone-grafts

Unification of bone is encouraged by homoeopathic *Symphytum*, as with *fractures*.

Bone spicule – *see* Sequestrum

Borax

Homeopathic sodium borate. An important remedy for the treatment of oral *candidosis*. It is also frequently useful in the treatment of *aphthous ulcers*, especially where the **susceptible typology** is appropriate: nervous, timid, very sensitive to loud noises, dread of downward motion (e.g. descent in an aircraft).

Breath, offensive or foul – *see* Halitosis

Bruxism & Bruxomania

Tooth grinding or clenching in adults is invariably associated with psychological disturbances, and may occur in the waking hours (bruxomania) or during sleep (bruxism). The psychological factors may be circumstantial or related to personality. Undoubtedly, the simplest approach is to use the *Bach flower remedies*. Otherwise, constitutional remedies are required. *Podophyllum, Zincum metallicum* and *Cannabis indica* are said to be frequently indicated, according to typology. In children, where the origin is less likely to be purely psychological, *Belladonna, Cina, Phytolacca* and *Bacillinum* are worthy of consideration.

Bryonia (Bryonia alba)*

Homoeopathic white bryony. A remedy for the relief of *fracture* pain, *pulpitis*, trigeminal *neuralgia* and *xerostomia*. With regard to pain in general, it is indicated where this is < movement, < the least touch, > local heat, > rest, and > strong pressure on the affected part. The typical pain is acute, piercing and lancinating. Bryonia is predominantly (though not exclusively) a right-sided remedy.

   Susceptible typology: irritable, easily annoyed, dark, robust, well-fed, < heat (except for local pains, which are > heat), > cold, great thirst with dry mouth (especially during a fever).

Fig. 9. Bryonia

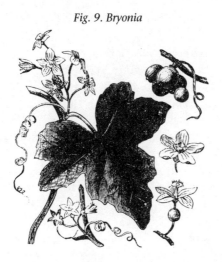

Bulimia nervosa – see Anorexia nervosa & bulimia nervosa

Burning mouth syndrome (BMS)

This is a burning sensation of the mouth without any visible abnormality of the oral mucosa. It is more common in women, with a peak incidence in the 40–50 year-old group. The most common site for the sensation is the tongue, followed by the palate and upper alveolar ridge, the lips, and the lower alveolar ridge. Less commonly, it occurs in the throat, buccal mucosa and floor of the mouth. The possible causative factors are numerous. These include: deficiency states (*iron, folate, vitamin B1, vitamin B2, vitamin B6, vitamin B12*), *diabetes mellitus* (uncontrolled or undiagnosed), oral *candidosis* (including *denture sore mouth*), *xerostomia*, poor denture design, psychological states (with or without tooth clenching or tongue thrusting habits) and menopausal syndromes. *Allergy* to dental materials, food or preservatives is relevant to only a minority of cases.

However, despite various investigations, including blood tests and attempts to identify candidosis, psychological approaches, the prescription of psychogenic drugs, denture adjustments and blind trials of vitamins B1, B2 or B6, a large number of cases persist and present themselves to the homoeopathist. Strangely enough, many sufferers (especially women over 40 years of age), despite apparently normal vitamin B12 levels, respond well to injections of that vitamin (hydroxocobalamin 1000mcg weekly, intramuscularly or deep subcutaneously), whereas oral supplementation frequently fails. In menopausal cases, *evening primrose oil* may also be helpful. Again, in cases associated with the menopause, key homoeopathic remedies are *Lachesis, Natrum muriaticum, Pulsatilla* and *Sepia*, prescribed according to their constitutional indications. The same remedies may be also indicated in non-menopausal cases. Other key remedies to be considered in general are *Arsenicum album, Phosphorus* and *Sulphur. Iris versicolor* may be helpful in cases with a strong history of migraine or migrainous *neuralgia*. Where either oral candidosis or xerostomia is present, homoeopathy may also be of service. Where there are distinct disturbances of the psyche, the use of the *Bach flower remedies* should not be forgotten.

Burns, instrument

'Hypercal' (*Hypericum* and *Calendula*) cream or ointment should be applied immediately. Alternatively, apply the oily contents of a *vitamin E* capsule.

C

Calarea group of remedies

This includes *Calarea carbonica, Calcarea fluorica, Calcarea phosphorica* and *Calcarea renalis*. Their importance from the dental point of view is that they all have some influence on calcium metabolism, and thus are collectively of great relevance to the correction of disorders of bone and teeth, and predispositions to *calculus* formation in the orofacial region.

Calcarea carbonica (Calcarea ostrearum)*

Homoeopathic oyster shell (impure calcium carbonate from the middle layer). Useful in some cases of *acromegaly, epulis*, delayed *eruption, mouth-breathing, ranula*, chronic *gingivitis* and *periodontitis*, and recurrent *caries*. It is sometimes employed in mild *pulpitis*, especially where a toothache < cold air follows a deep filling. **Susceptible typology:** short, fat, stubby hands, brachycephalic, broad (square) anterior teeth, flat palate, wide dental arches, absence of crowding, retarded eruption, *tongue* indented, easily discouraged, slow to get going in any task (but then gathers momentum), fearful, chilly, inactive, an intense desire for eggs, prone to urinary and gall-bladder stone formation, children with big sweaty heads.

See also *Endodontics*.

Calcarea fluorica*

Homoeopathic calcium fluoride. Useful in the treatment of recurrent *sprains, dislocation* of the jaw, *exostoses, fibrous dysplasia, haemangiomata, salivary gland* disorders (including *sialectasis*), *osteopetrosis*, chronic *periodontitis* and predisposition to *caries*. it may also be useful in *orthodontics* to assist movement of the teeth. **Susceptible typology:** small or medium build, dolicocephalic, mandibular or maxillary prognathism, obvious asymmetry of face and dental arches, small and overcrowded teeth with poor and grey enamel, teeth erupt out of normal sequence, delayed *eruption*, slender bones, laxness of articulations (carrying angle of elbow in excess of 180°), scoliosis, children lack concentration and discipline, generally < changes in climate.

Calcarea phosphorica*

Homoeopathic calcium phosphate. A remedy for the facilitation of *orthodontic* movement of teeth, the predisposition to *caries, fractures,* tonsillar enlargement with *mouth-breathing, gingivitis* of puberty, *Paget's disease, osteogenesis imperfecta* and *fibrous dysplasia* (including Albright's syndrome). **Susceptible typology:** tall, thin, elegant, long eye lashes, narrow face, well-arched palate, teeth long and narrow (and yellowish), tendency to crowding, precocious or delayed *eruption*, tendency to exostoses, precocious puberty, easily tired by intellectual work but intelligent, emotional instability, agitated, sensitive, sentimental, timid, prefers to be left alone, desires preserved and salty meats, < change in climate.

Calcarea renalis

Homoeopathic preparation of calcium urate renal calculus. A remedy for reducing dental *calculus* formation, sometimes inducing its loss, especially in subjects prone to gout.

Calciferol – see **Vitamin D**

Calcium

An adequate dietetic intake of calcium is necessary for the proper development of teeth and bone, and maintenance of the latter. Regulation of calcium metabolism is partially determined by satisfactory levels of *vitamin D*. Diminishing oestrogen levels occurring at the menopause favour the loss of calcium from the bones and thus osteoporosis. It would seem likely that calcium deficient diets, lack of vitamin D or menopausal changes are, to some degree, contributory to periodontal bone destruction or the loss of the *prosthetic* ridge. Studies have suggested that combined calcium and vitamin D supplementation may be useful in reducing alveolar bone loss in those who wear dentures. It may also turn out that calcium-rich diets (e.g. where there is a good intake of canned fish or dairy products), combined with *evening primrose oil*, may be helpful in retarding periodontal and alveolar ridge bone loss in menopausal or postmenopausal females.

See also *Fluoridation; Fracture, jaw; Periodontitis, chronic.*

Calculus, dental (Tartar)

In order to retard the formation of dental calculus, try *Fragaria* 6 twice daily for some months. Should this fail, consider *Calcarea renalis* 6 twice daily. Either remedy may also induce the actual loss of existing calculus. Both are generally suitable for administration in conjunction with other remedies in cases of chronic *gingivitis* or periodontitis.

Calculus, salivary – see **Salivary calculus**

Calendula (Calendula officinalis)

A botanic remedy adopted by homoeopathy, though seldom used in its potentised form. The mother tincture is prepared from the leaves and flowers of the marigold, and is applied topically in either aqueous dilution, or as a 5% ointment or cream. Calendula officinalis belongs to the same family of plants (Compositae) as *Arnica* and *Bellis perennis*, and is, like these, a great vulnerary. Unlike Arnica, it is suitable for intraoral use and may be applied to broken skin, provided that it is first diluted. Its important application is with regard to incisional or lacerated wounds and tooth extraction. In this respect, it has four major properties: the promotion of healing of epithelial tissues, the prevention of infection (by virtue of its antiseptic qualities), the induction of haemostasis (an action similar to that of Arnica and Bellis perennis) and the reduction of pain and discomfort. It is valuable also in the treatment of *abrasions*, where it is usually applied as an ointment or cream. Aqueous dilutions are best administered as hot as can be safely tolerated. For external use, a dilution of 1 in 20 is suitable. Fomentations may be repeatedly applied to areas of lacerated skin, even if a compound *fracture* is present beneath. Calendula is of great service in traumatic and general *oral surgery*. For intraoral use, about 30 drops of Calendula Ø should be added to 500ml of hot water. This may be used as a *mouthwash*, or gauze may be soaked in the solution, and the fomentation pressed against the tooth socket or wound. In the case of an extraction, the fomentation can be held in place by the approximation of the jaws. Mouthwashes should be repeated 3–4 times daily, until full healing occurs. Some prefer to add an additional 30 drops of *Hypericum* Ø to each 500ml of water, in order to favour the repair of damaged nerves.

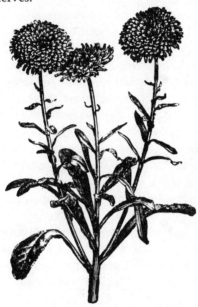

Fig. 10. Calendula

Cancer – *see* **Tumours & cysts**

Cancrum oris (Noma)

Gangrene of the cheek, occurring principally in children. This serious condition is now essentially restricted to impoverished countries, being related to severe malnutrition in conjunction with a major infection, such as measles or tuberculosis. The organisms responsible are similar to those of *ANUG*. Rapid unilateral gangrenous destruction of the cheek may progress to *osteomyelitis* of the jaw, and death by *septicaemia* or bronchopneumonia. Antibiotics are often unavailable. Treatment should commence with *Kali chloricum* 30 and *Pyrogen* 30, given conjointly twice daily; preferably with a dose of *Anthracinum* 30 being give at midday. Where Kali chloricum is unavailable, *Mercurius corrosivus* 30 may be sub-stituted (this may, indeed, by the only remedy available). Obviously, treatment will be facilitated by the correction of nutritional deficiencies (especially those of *vitamin C* and *zinc*) where possible.

Candidosis, oral (Candidiasis, oral)

The mere presence of candida species within the mouth is not necessarily indicative of disease, since about 2 persons out of 5 harbour these organisms as part of their normal oral microflora. Whereas there are a number of different species of intraoral candida, and all have the potential to produce the infection termed 'oral candidosis', the dominant offender is Candida albicans. Predisposing factors are numerous: *iron* deficiency, *vitamin B2* deficiency, *vitamin B12* deficiency, *vitamin C* deficiency, *zinc* deficiency, excessive sugar intake, malnutrition, *pellagra*, infancy, old age, poorly controlled *diabetes mellitus, agranulocytosis, AIDS, leukaemia, hypothyroidism, xerostomia, pregnancy,* drug therapies (including *antibiotics,* immunosuppressive agents, cytotoxic agents and *corticosteroids*) and *prosthetic* or *orthodontic* appliances. Various types of oral candidosis are described:

(1) Acute pseudomembranous candidosis (thrush). This is characterised by soft creamy white or yellowish plaques, which can be wiped away to reveal an erythematous mucosa. It commonly affects neonates, the elderly, those with agranulocytosis or AIDS, and those undergoing antibiotic or steroid therapy. A chronic pseudomembranous type also occurs.

(2) Acute erythematous (atrophic) candidosis. This is often a painful condition, unlike other types of oral candidosis, and is seen in association with antibiotic or steroid therapy, and AIDS. The oral mucosa is erythematous.

(3) Chronic erythematous (atrophic) candidosis. This is alternatively termed 'denture sore mouth' and is an erythematous mucosal condition related to coverage of the oral mucosa by Prosthetic or upper removable orthodontic appliances.

(4) Chronic plaque-like/nodular (hyperplastic) candidosis, alternatively termed 'candidal leukoplakia'. Hyperplastic epithelial changes occur, characteristically (but not exclusively) in the commissure regions of the buccal mucosa, presenting clinically as speckled white patches. Occasionally, premalignant or malignant changes occur in the lesions, particularly at the commissure site.

(5) Candida-associated *angular cheilitis*.

Investigations include scrape, smear, oral rinse and biopsy. Oral candidosis may, of course, be associated with candidosis elsewhere in the body (e.g. vagina, intestines).

In treatment, any obvious deficiency states should be corrected (iron, vitamin B2, zinc, etc.). Other underlying disorders also require attention. A diet which excludes most overt sugar (sweets, chocolates, honey, cakes, biscuits, drinks with added sugar, etc.) and crisps should be instituted; although fruits, natural fruit juices and dried fruits need only be excluded in resistant cases. Garlic or garlic supplements should be taken freely. The key remedy for most intraoral cases is *Borax* 30–200, given two or three times daily. Should this fail, consider either *Kali muriaticum* 30 two or three times daily, or Candida albicans nosode 6 twice daily (indeed, the latter may be given in conjunction with other remedies). Such systemic treatment may be complemented with *mouthwashes*, ointments or creams containing extracts of *Aloe vera, Berberis vulgaris* or *Hydrastis canadensis* (or combinations of these), all three of which (as with garlic) have anticandidal properties. *Caprylic acid* added to a cream or ointment may also prove to be useful. Resistant cases may require homoeopathic constitutional treatment.

Tea tree oil is also worthy of mention. A cotton-bud impregnated with one drop of this oil of relatively low toxicity may be used to treat infantile thrush. The mouth is briefly and thoroughly swabbed. One or two treatments (12 hours apart) should suffice. A similar approach may be tried in adult cases of oral candidosis (? all types), using 2–3 drops per cotton-bud.

See also *Median rhomboid glossitis*.

Cannabis indica

Homoeopathic hashish. A remedy for *bruxism* or bruxomania in patients of the appropriate typology. **Susceptible typology:** loquacious, cannot finish a sentence, confused, fearful, excessive laughter.

Caprylic acid

A short-chain fatty acid, known chemically as octanoic acid, and found naturally in coconut oil and breast milk. Most organic fatty acids are fungicidal, but caprylic acid is particularly effective in *candidosis*. It mimics the fatty acids produced by the normal bowel flora, which are a major component of the defensive system against candida infection. Caprylic acid is usually given internally, but may be incorporated in an ointment or cream base for local use.

Car-sickness, patients arriving with – *see* Zingiber

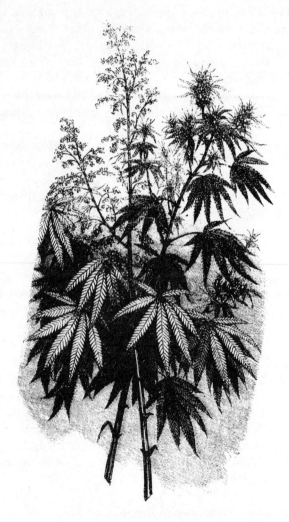

Fig. 11. Cannabis indica

Carbo vegetabilis*

Homoeopathic wood charcoal. Although a constitutional remedy in its own right, its principal application in dental surgery is the treatment of sudden *collapse* of serious origin, such as myocardial infarction, irrespective of susceptible typology. For this purpose, it is generally given in a potency of 30c, but may be used higher. It may be helpful in cases of *xerostomia*, where the typological indications are appropriate. **Susceptible typology:** elderly, feeble, tired, pale or cyanotic, dyspeptic, internal burning and external cold, desires to be fanned, aversion to fat and meat, aversion to milk, prone to varicose ulcers, < heat and humidity, < alcohol.

Carbolicum acidum (Acidum carbolicum)

Homoeopathic phenol. It is indicated by the presence of severe acute pains (which are usually lancinating or burning), which appear suddenly, last a short time and disappear abruptly. It is thus of service in some cases of facial *neuralgia*.

Carcinoma – see Tumours & cysts

Caries, predisposition to dental

Despite the apparent success of *fluoridation* programmes, there is now a world-wide resurgence of caries in the 5 year-old group of developed countries; and it would appear that the same will be found in 12 year-olds. This has not been explained. Hence, homoeopathy may once again be applied to the problem. For early and rapid decay of the deciduous dentition, consider *Kreasotum* 6–12 twice daily as the prime treatment (this remedy may also be indicated in some adult cases). For the pre-disposition to caries in general, observe the dominant morphology of the face and intraoral structures, and select *Calcarea carbonica, Calcarea fluorica* or *Calcarea phosphorica*, according to the indications given under these headings. Where a decision based upon the orofacial morphology alone is difficult, then the more general aspects of the three susceptible typologies must be taken into account in order to select the correct remedy. The selected remedy should be given initially in a potency of 6–12c twice daily. Prescriptions of Kreasotum or the Calcareae must usually be given for many months. The treatment may be fortified by the infrequent use of *Bacillinum*. However, since the use of this nosode requires some degree of experience, newcomers to homoeopathy should take advice on this matter from the professional homoeopathist. The combination of chronic *periodontitis* and high caries rate is more indicative of *Staphysagria* 6–12 twice daily. The combination of *root caries* and severe chronic periodontitis suggests *Thuja* 6–12 twice daily. It should be noted that some cases of gross caries are associated with *xerostomia* (dry mouth), and these may require different remedial treatment.

Carpal tunnel syndrome

I mention this for the benefit of the dental surgeon so afflicted, since, in many cases, operation can be avoided. Certainly, *osteopathy* and more particularly *chiropractic* are highly beneficial. The main focus of attention will be the reduction of thoracic and cervical vertebral displacements, which are often contributory to the generation of the syndrome. Additionally, *vitamin B6* 50mg three times daily should be taken (this dose must not be exceeded).

Causticum*

Homeopathic. Prepared by distilling a mixture of slaked lime and potassium sulphate. Of great importance in the treatment of lower motor neurone *facial nerve palsy* in most susceptible typologies. Causticum is to motor nerves as *Hypericum* is to sensory. Indicated in some cases of *median rhomboid glossitis* and facial *neuralgia*. **Susceptible typology:** thin, tired, very chilly, intense need for sympathy, extremely sensitive to the problems of others, quarrelsome, children cry easily and are afraid of going to bed alone, > heat and humidity, desires smoked and salted meats, burning sensations with tenderness.

Cellulitis, acute

Severe spreading infections of the orofacial tissues are the occasional result of dental sepsis, but also may occur following trauma. Ludwig's angina, stemming from an infected mandibular tooth and perhaps the most dangerous, is relatively rare. Nowadays, since acute cellulitis is a potentially fatal condition, it is difficult, from the medicolegal point of view, not to recommend antibiotics, Nevertheless, homoeopathic treatment is fully justified where the patient refuses to take orthodox medication, where antibiotics are ineffective or where they are unavailable (as in many developing countries). The key remedy is undoubtedly *Belladonna* 30–200 given every 2–6 hours. This is well-indicated where the patient is very thirsty during the fever. Where the patient is thirstless during the fever, *Apis mellifica* 30–200 with the same repetition, may be better indicated. The swelling of the Belladonna type is not so

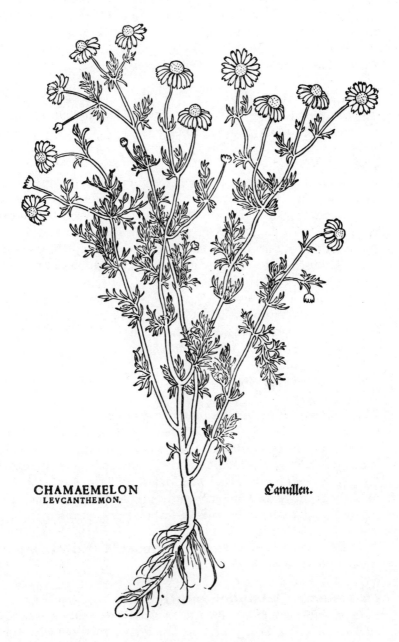

CHAMAEMELON
LEVCANTHEMON.

Camillen.

Fig. 12. Chamomilla

profound as the Apis type, and very red. The Apis swelling tends to be gross, and the skin overlying it is more of a rose colour. An alternative to either Belladonna or Apis is *Myristica* 30 every 1–6 hours.

Cementum, sensitive – see Cervical sensitivity

Cervical sensitivity

Admirable results have been obtained by applying undiluted *Plantago* Ø 1–3 times daily to the sensitive area.

Chamomilla*

Homoeopathic chamomile. In dentistry, primarily a remedy for *teething* infants and fractious *children*. Also indicated in some cases of acute dental *anxiety* in adults, *aerodontalgia*, *pulpitis*, median fissure of the *lip*, *median rhomboid glossitis* and *halitosis*. It is sometimes used to treat systemic or psychic reactions to local *anaesthesia*. **Susceptible typology:**

(1) Children: tired, disagreeable, capricious, throws away what is given, one cheek red and the other pale.

(2) Adults: nervous, extremely pain sensitive, normally civil but angry and rude when in pain, aversion to or intense desire for coffee, generally > heat but toothache > cold water (< hot food).

See also *Pain threshold, low*.

Chancre – see Syphilis

Cheek biting, recurrent (Stomatitis artefacta)

Recurrent cheek biting in both children and adults is usually a manifestation of psychological disturbance. Treatment of the psyche involves the use of *Bach flower remedies* or homoeopathic constitutional remedies. Local treatments for the *bitten cheek*, or any *aphthous ulcers* produced by biting, may also be used simultaneously. In children, recurrent cheek biting may produce the appearance of a white *sponge naevus*.

Cheilitis – see Angular cheilitis; Exfoliative cheilitis; Lip, median fissure of lower

Cheiranthus (Cheiranthus cheiri)

Homoeopathic common wallflower. A remedy for acute *trismus* associated with dental *abscess, pericoronitis, craniomandibular dysfunction* or *oral surgery*. It is also a remedy for pericoronitis itself, in the absence of trismus. A leading symptom to its use is 'nose obstructed at night as a result of cutting of wisdom teeth'.

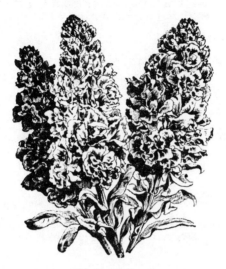

Fig. 13. Cheiranthus

Chickenpox (Varicella)

This is caused by Varicella zoster virus infection, as is *herpes zoster* and *Ramsay-Hunt syndrome*. Apart from the characteristic vesiculopustular rash of the skin, oral *ulcers*, 2–4mm in diameter, may appear in the faucial and palatal regions. *Mouthwashes* of aqueous dilutions of *Calendula* or *Propolis* Ø may be used several times daily. Fundamental treatment of the condition usually involves the use of potentised *Antimonium tartaricum, Rhus toxicodendron* or *Sulphur*.

Children, fractious

The main remedy here is *Chamomilla* 30, preferably given morning and evening on the day before and one hour prior to the procedure; otherwise, every 15 minutes until the child is calmed. Its indications are: whining restlessness, spiteful, oversensitive to pain, cross, irritable desire to be carried or petted (which >), uncooperative, throws away toys or objects given to calm. *Cina* 30 has similar indications, but the child does not want to be touched, carried, or even looked at. The dose repetition is as for Chamomilla.

See also *Pain threshold, low*.

China (Cinchona officinalis)

Homoeopathic Peruvian bark. A remedy occasionally indicated in dental *haemorrhage*, especially if accompanied by blurred vision, buzzing in the ear, great weakness, and a desire to be fanned (< heat). Also useful for general weakness and debility following an episode of haemorrhage.

Chipped tooth – *see* Traumatised tooth

Chiropractic

A group of methods of manipulation of use in the treatment of *craniomandibular dysfunction*, migraine or migrainous *neuralgia* and *carpal tunnel syndrome*.

Christmas disease (Haemophilia B) – *see* Haemophilia

Chrysanthemum parthenium – *see* Feverfew

Cina

Homoeopathic wormseed. Useful to calm certain types of fractious *children*, and an important remedy for threadworms, irrespective of susceptible typology. Indicated in some cases of *bruxism* in children. **Susceptible typology:** sullen, disagreeable, irritable, throws away what is given, does not want to be touched or looked at (compare *Chamomilla*), cries as soon as looked at or picked up, rings around eyes, yawns constantly, agitated sleep, clenches teeth at night, prone to threadworms.

See also *Bruxism & bruxomania*.

Cinchona officinalis – *see* China

Cinnabaris

Homoeopathic mercury sulphide. Indicated in some cases of trigeminal *neuralgia*, with violent periorbital lancinating pains radiating from the lacrimal orifice to the temple, accompanied by redness of the eye and pain on the least contact; < humidity, < extremes of temperature, < at night.

Cistus canadensis

Homoeopathic ice plant. A remedy for chronic *gingivitis* and *periodontitis*, where the gums are thin, friable and bleed easily. Also a remedy for malignant disease of the glands of the neck, when they are stony hard. **Susceptible typology:** patients who are extremely sensitive to cold air, mouth and saliva feel cold, prone to cervical lymphadenopathy ('scrofulous').

Cleidocranial dysostosis

A congenital condition which neither affects the intellect nor longevity. Ossification of the cranial bones is defective and there is partial development or entire absence of the clavicles. Recurrent *dislocation* of the TMJ may occur in some cases.

Clematis erecta

Homoeopathic upright virgin's bower. A remedy for *toothache* < lying down and > for holding cold water in the mouth (compare *Chamomilla* and *Coffea cruda*). Sometimes used in the treatment of *pulpitis*.

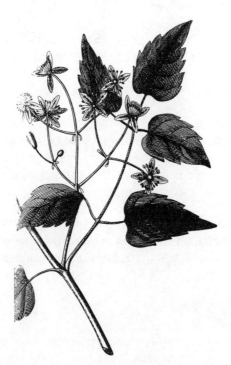

Fig. 14. Clematis erecta

Clove oil (Oil of cloves/Oleum Caryophylli)

Obtained by distillation of cloves. A traditional botanic treatment for *toothache* related to a lost filling or carious cavity. It is introduced via a cotton-wool plug. Contact with the oral mucosa may lead to irritation and inflammation, which may resemble an *aspirin burn*. The treatment is similar.

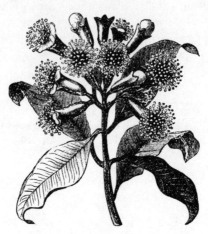

Fig. 15. Cloves

Cluster headache – *see* Neuralgia, (periodic) migrainous

Coccus cacti

Homoeopathic cochineal (the female insect). A remedy which, in its potentised form, assists in the expulsion of foreign bodies from the conjunctival sac, and thus helps to prevent the development of *conjunctivitis*.

Coeliac disease

This may be associated with *aphthous* ulceration of the mouth. This often improves dramatically with gluten exclusion, but resistant cases require assessment of *folate* levels, with appropriate supplementation where necessary.

See also *Vitamin E.*

Coenzyme Q10

Also known as ubiquinone-50. Coenzyme Q10 is a vital catalyst to the provision of energy for all cells. A common feature of chronic *gingivitis* or *periodontitis* is a local deficiency of this substance, which may be due

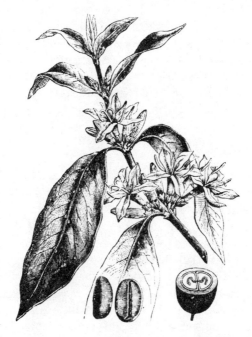

Fig. 16. Coffea cruda

to the condition itself or may be additionally associated, in a proportion of cases, with a generalised coenzyme Q10 deficiency state. Results have been encouraging in improving the periodontium with internally administered doses, generally 30mg once daily (range: 20–50 mg daily, according to response). At present, it is not recommended for use during pregnancy and in lactation. Side effects are rare and only occur in less than 1% of cases. These include: gastric discomfort, nausea, loss of appetite and diarrhoea. Those who are particularly interested in this valuable addition to the dental therapeutic armamentarium should ask for the leaflet 'Coenzyme Q10' by Dr Leonard Mervyn, supplied free of charge by Lamberts Healthcare Ltd., 1 Lamberts Road, Tunbridge Wells, Kent TN2 3EQ, England. This contains valuable references to the research work carried out to date in the area of periodontology.

Coffea (Coffea cruda)*

Homoeopathic Arabic coffee seeds (unroasted). Useful in some cases of acute dental *anxiety, aerodontalgia,* and *pulpitis* alleviated by holding cold water in the mouth and < heat (compare *Chamomilla* and *Clematis erecta*). As the water warms in the mouth, so the pain returns. These phenomena are probably related to the presence of pulpal gases, which expand with heat or contract with cold. **Susceptible typology:** nervous, intelligent, overactive, hyperaesthesia of all senses, hypersensitive to pain, mind full of thoughts, poor sleep, easily overstimulated by pleasant events, generally < cold but toothache > cold. The Coffea patient is very sensitive to noise, even 'decent' music in the surgery, and demands that it should be turned off.

See also *Pain threshold, low*.

Cold sore – *see* Herpes labialis

Colds & influenza, prevention of

The dental surgeon is particularly exposed to the risk of contracting these from the infected patient. Adequate *zinc* and *vitamin C* levels should be maintained by diet or supplementation. Additionally *Oscillococcinum* 200 should be taken as a single dose on alternate days as a preventative. Should symptoms develop, *Aconite* 30 may be taken immediately, together with *Zingiber* Ø 20 drops in a little water. Both should be repeated ever 4 hours until symptoms remit.

See also *Thrombocytopenia*.

Collapse, sudden

Apart from normal first-aid measures, homoeopathy may be of great assistance. For a simple faint, give *Bach* Rescue Remedy 3 drops every minute until recovery occurs. Good old-fashioned *smelling salts* are a sensible alternative or additional therapy. Some prefer to give Veratrum album 30 (homoeopathic white hellebore). More serious cases (e.g. CVA, myocardial infarction) require *Carbo vegetabilis* 30 (liquid potency) every 5 minutes until help arrives. This remedy may be life-saving. If there is any doubt about the nature of the collapse, always give Carbo vegetabilis, sometimes termed 'the homoeopathic corpse reviver'.

Concussion

Where concussion complicates traumatic cases, or where the head has been severely jarred without concussion, give *Natrum sulphuricum* 30 4-hourly.

Concussion, pulpal – *see* Pulpitis; Traumatised tooth

Condyloma acuminatum
This is a sessile papillomatous lesion of the oral or genital regions, usually found in groups. Oral lesions generally occur as a result of orogenital contact in either heterosexuals or homosexuals. The occurrence of these in children may be suggestive of sexual abuse, but the appearance of the lesion at any age may be clinically identical to squamous cell *papilloma*, which is of non-venereal origin. For non-surgical treatment, see *Papillomavirus lesions, human.*

Conjunctivitis, acute
To assist the expulsion of foreign particles (such as amalgam slurry and tooth fragments) from the conjunctival sac, take *Coccus cacti* 30 every 10 minutes or so. Established mild acute conjunctivitis may be treated with *Euphrasia* 30 three times daily. More severe acute conjunctivitis, with much purulent discharge, may require *Argentum nitricum* 30 three times daily. Any case may benefit from the additional use, instilled 3–6 times daily, of the following drop formula: Triple Rose Water 5ml, distilled water 5 ml, Euphrasia Ø 3 drops.

Contraceptives, oral – *see* Folate; Vitamin B6

Corticosteroids
Therapy with steroid inhalers may be associated with *angina bullosa haemorrhagica* and oral *candidosis*. Other types of corticosteroid therapy are also associated with oral candidosis.

Cost-effectiveness of homoeopathy
One great virtue of homoeopathic remedies is their relatively low cost compared with orthodox alternatives in the field of oral medicine. Refer to the article by H.W. Feldhaus, British Homoeopathic Journal, January 1993, Vol. 82, pp. 22–28.

Costen's syndrome – *see* Craniomandibular dysfunction

Coxsackieviruses
These give rise to *hand, foot & mouth disease* and *herpangina*, both with oral manifestations.
　　See also *Salivary glands, viral infections of.*

Cramp

Episodes of cramp in the legs or arms may be treated with *Cuprum metallicum* 30 every 10 minutes. Cramps may sometimes be caused by a low salt diet or excessive *zinc* supplementation.

Craniomandibular dysfunction (TMJ dysfunction syndrome)

One aspect of *facial pain*, which goes by a variety of names, including Costen's syndrome and facial arthromyalgia. In this condition the TMJ is anatomically, radiographically and pathologically normal. The key diagnostic subjective and objective symptoms, which may be present either unilaterally or bilaterally (all of which may not be exhibited), are: preauricular pain, which may radiate to the mandibular, maxillary, temporal or occipital areas, and which may undergo acute exacerbation; headaches; limitation of jaw opening, including frank *trismus*; difficulty in chewing; tenderness over the TMJ and of the muscles of mastication; and audible or palpable clicking of the TMJ. This syndrome must be distinguished from disease of the *TMJ*, *tetanus*, oromandibular *dystonia* and intraoral infection, such as dental *abscess* and *pericoronitis*.

Mechanical therapies include the provision of dentures, the correction of mallocclusion and acrylic splints (bite-plates). Nevertheless, many cases fail treatment. Where psychological causes are apparent, especially in cases of *bruxism* or bruxomania, then the use of either *Bach flower remedies* or constitutional remedies is indicated. *Staphysagria* should be thought of in cases of stifled vexation, or where the complaint has arisen from a psychological 'stab in the back' or sexual abuse. Some appear to be a manifestation of *mercury toxicity* or sensitivity to chrome-cobalt, and respond to the removal of amalgams or the provision of gold alloy prostheses respectively. Even so, it is apparent that many practitioners fail to realise that a large proportion of cases are related to vertebral displacement, requiring the services of *osteopathy* or *chiropractic*. In this respect, the reduction of both thoracic and cervical displacements should be a prime approach in the treatment of most sufferers. A particular area of attention, often missed, is C7/T1, which is best dealt with by chiropractic manipulation. Sometimes, relief, albeit partial, is almost instant. In order to fortify the effect, *acupuncture* is particularly helpful. Although there are many local and remote points which might be needled, a key point is Stomach 6, situated at the angle of the jaw. The needle should be inserted perpendicularly to the skin until the mandible is contacted, not manipulated in any way, and not left in for more than 3 minutes. This is often a most helpful technique. My fashion is to repeat vertebral manipulation (if indicated) and acupuncture at weekly intervals until significant improvement has occurred. Attempts to find 'specific' remedies for craniomandibular dysfunction have not been particularly fruitful, although *Hypericum* 30 three times daily is useful in some cases, and *Cheiranthus* 30 two or three times daily may relieve frank trismus. Fischer recommends *Magnesia phosphorica* 30 (or higher) several times daily to reduce muscle spasm which is > heat. As he points out, only the muscular component of the disorder is usually relieved by this prescription. *Zincum phosphoricum* 30 three times daily is sometimes useful in individuals suffering from mental exhaustion. The old favourite *Rhus toxicodendron* 30, three times daily, is to be considered where there is clicking or cracking of the TMJ, the jaw is especially stiff in the morning and loosens with use (talking, eating, posturing) during the day, and improves with the application of heat or in warm weather (< damp, cold weather). Without these individualising features, the remedy is unlikely to help. Otherwise, a better approach is to prescribe again on the basis of the individuality of the case, and consider such remedies as would normally be considered in cases of migrainous *neuralgia*. Indeed, there are some instances where the differentiation between craniomandibular dysfunction and migrainous neuralgia is most difficult. Since, however, there is a common thread of manipulative, acupuncture and homoeopathic therapies with regard to both disorders, a combined approach is often successful, even though a definite orthodox diagnosis has not been made.

See also *Facial pain, atypical; Tension headache.*

Crataegus
Mother tincture of hawthorn berries. A botanic adopted by homoeopathy primarily for the treatment of the heart affected by coronary atherosclerosis; yet, it has no effect on the normal heart. In dentistry, its sole use is in the treatment of diarrhoea following the administration of *antibiotics*.

CREST syndrome – *see* **Scleroderma**

Cretinism – *see* **Hypothyroidism**

Fig. 17. Crataegus

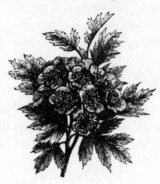

Crohn's disease

Oral lesions are not uncommon in this condition, and may even precede any involvement of the terminal ileum. They include: *aphthous ulcers* (20%), *angular cheilitis*, full width *gingivitis*, lip swelling, mucosal tags, oedema of the buccal mucosa, *epidermolysis bullosa* acquisita and *pyostomatitis vegetans*. Local treatments of lesions are applicable with *Myrrh* or *Propolis*, and injections of *vitamin B12* are indicated in cases of vitamin B12 malabsorption. Otherwise homoeopathic constitutional and antimiasmatic treatment should be administered.

　　See also *Orofacial granulomatosis*.

Cuprum metallicum

Homoeopathic copper. A great remedy for muscular *cramp*, especially in the elderly, often used preventatively.

Cuts

Use potentised *Arnica* internally to control bleeding and bruising. Use *Calendula* cream externally to promote healing.

Cyst – *see* Tumours & cysts

Cyst, periapical – *see* Endodontics

Cytomegalovirus – *see* Salivary glands, viral infections of

D

Dental abscess – *see* **Abscess, dental**

Dental caries – *see* **Caries, predisposition to dental**

Dentifrices – *see* **Toothpastes, homoeopathic & botanic**

Dentinogenesis imperfecta – *see* **Osteogenesis imperfecta**

Denture granuloma

This is essentially *scar* tissue in response to trauma from the flange of a *prosthetic* appliance. Reduction of size occurs after correction of the prosthetic defect. That which remains after one month is best removed surgically, with the normal homoeopathic precautions indicated for *oral surgery* in general.

Denture sore mouth – *see* **Candidosis, oral; Prosthetics, dental**

Dentures, problems associated with – *see* **Prosthetics, dental**

Dermatitis herpetiformis

A rare chronic disease, with the highest prevalence in Scandinavia. It is characterised by pruritic papules, herpetiform vesicles and papulo-vesicles, mainly on the skin of the elbows, posterior neck, scalp, knees and buttocks. Oral lesions occur in the form of erosions and bullae, and these occasionally precede dermal manifestations. Some considerable improvement may be derived from dietary exclusion of gluten. Local oral treatments, as for *aphthous ulcers*, may be helpful. Constitutional therapy is required for the underlying disorder.

See also *Ulcers*.

Dermatitis, perioral – *see* **Perioral dermatitis**

Diabetes mellitus

Oral lesions associated with this disorder include: oral *candidosis, angular cheilitis, burning mouth syndrome, gingivitis, periodontitis and sialosis*. *Lichenoid reactions* may occur in association with the administration of oral hypoglycaemic drugs. *Sialorrhoea* is a symptom of diabetic autonomic neuropathy, and may improve with the administration of *evening primrose oil* (1–4g daily).

Dislocation, TMJ

Immediately after reduction of an isolated dislocation of the TMJ, *Arnica* 30 should be given three or four times daily for several days. Recurrent dislocation, however, is another problem. Here, *Calcarea fluorica* 6–12 or *Strontium carbonicum* 30, given twice daily for several months, may assist cases with damage to the ligamentous tissues of the joint. Some cases are associated with hypermobility of the joints in general, which may occur in people essentially 'normal' in other respects, or in cases of *Ehrlers-Danlos syndrome, osteogenesis imperfecta, cleidocranial dysostosis* and *Marfan's syndrome*. Those with general hypermobility of the joints are best treated with *Calcarea fluorica*. If psychological conditions are associated, the use of the *Bach flower remedies* or constitutional remedies may be indicated. It is important to distinguish recurrent dislocation from oromandibular *dystonia*.

Dislocation, tooth – *see* Reimplantation

Dispensary, the dental – *see* Appendix 1

Dry mouth – *see* Xerostomia

Dry socket (Infected tooth socket)

Local treatment includes dressings soaked in an equal mixture of *Propolis* Ø and *Plantago* Ø, and the use of *Myrrh* mouthwashes (Ø 5ml plus water 45ml). Where there is throbbing pain, give *Belladonna* 30 hourly. Otherwise, Fischer considers *Ruta* to be the prime remedy in the treatment of dry socket, to be used at the outset of most cases (30c hourly). He also feels that *Pyrogen* (30c two or three times daily) may be required additionally. Where the pain improves with cold water held in the mouth, consider *Chamomilla* 30–200 hourly; or, alternatively, *Coffea cruda* 30–200 or *Clematis erecta* 30. Where the pain is neither throbbing nor alleviated by cold water, or other remedies fail, consider *Hekla lava* 30 2-hourly. To assist in the expulsion of sequestra, give *Silicea* 6–12 three times daily.

The preoperative use of *Phosphorus*, to prevent excessive bleeding following extraction, is thought by some to increase the likelihood of dry socket.

Dyskeratosis congenita – see **Sponge naevus, white**

Dystonia, oromandibular

Dystonia is the term used to describe particular types of involuntary and abnormal movements and postures seen in a variety of neurological disorders. Oromandibular dystonia affects the tongue, mouth and jaw. The spasms may result in the mouth opening widely, sometimes with *dislocation*, or severe *trismus*. The most common type of dystonia is ITD or idiopathic torsion dystonia, probably associated with a biochemical abnormality of the basal ganglia of the brain, and often inherited. No other neurological deficits are discovered, and intellect is preserved. Secondary dystonia is associated with other neurological diseases (e.g. Parkinson's) or drug therapies (e.g. those used in schizophrenia). Dystonia may be confused with *craniomandibular dysfunction* and recurrent *dislocation* of the jaw. Surgical intervention in cases of recurrent dislocation should always be delayed until a neurologist skilled in the diagnosis of dystonia has been consulted. Oromandibular dystonia is most difficult to treat, although *acupuncture* and homoeopathy might achieve some partial alleviation. There is, in any event, 5–10% chance of remission, albeit temporary, with regard to ITD.

E

Ecthyma contagiosum (Orf)

This viral disease is contracted by contact with live or dead sheep, lambs, goats or kids, or indirectly via fomites. At the site of inoculation (which may be upon the face or neck) a lesion develops after an incubation period of 3–7 days. This is essentially a papule, some 1–4cm in diameter, covered with clear vesicles. These coalesce to form an umbilicated bulla, which then crusts over. This may take up to 8 weeks to heal, and there is regional enlargement of the lymph nodes. This lesion may be confused with a malignant tumour or tuberculosis. However, the extremely rapid development of the lesion and a history of contact with the relevant animals (farmers, butchers, vets, etc.) suggests the diagnosis. The key remedies for therapy are *Nitricum acidum, Rhus toxicodendron* and Orf nosode.

Ehlers-Danlos syndrome

This inherited disorder is of some importance to the dental surgeon. Its relevant characteristics are hypermobility of the joints in general; recurrent *dislocation* of the TMJ; skin fragility, associated with gaping wounds that are difficult to suture, leaving thin and spreading scars; excessive bruising after minor trauma; and protracted *haemorrhage* after dental extraction. Long-term *Calcarea fluorica* 6–12 twice daily may be helpful in controlling the disorder, and *Arnica* for both the prevention and treatment of haemorrhage and bruising should be considered.

Endocarditis – see Subacute bacterial endocarditis, prevention of

Endodontics

The sterilisation of root canals is best achieved by the use of paper points saturated with *Propolis* Ø. The administration of *Hepar sulph.* 6 three times daily is recommended throughout the course of endodontia in order to reduce periapical inflammation, but should be discontinued about 7 days after satisfactory occlusion of the root canal. Some cases, however, exhibit an annoying persistence of periapical tenderness and discomfort for many weeks or months after an apparently successful root canal filling. *Zinc* supplementation (adult dose: 15–30mg elemental zinc daily) and *Hepar sulph.* 30 twice daily are recommended. Others may require *Silicea* 6 twice daily. These secondary approaches are also justified in cases where permanent root filling cannot be performed because of frank and persistent periapical infection, despite apparently correct root canal sterilisation. Where a periapical cyst is suspected, *Hekla lava* 6 two or three times daily should be considered, with the hope of avoiding apicectomy or extraction (Silicea may also be considered secondarily in this respect). Apicectomy should always be accompanied by the routine use of *Arnica* and *Hypericum*, as for *oral surgery* in general (see also *Oral surgery, pain control after.*)

Where pain has been caused by apical penetration of a reamer, give *Ruta* 30–200, initially every 15–30 minutes as necessary.

It should be emphasised that the judicious use of remedies for *pulpitis* may preserve the vitality of the pulp. Furthermore, Fischer notes that the use of *Belladonna* initially, and later *Calcarea carbonica*, in some cases of inevitable pulpal necrosis, where they are properly indicated, removes the need for root-filling. Teeth treated in this manner sometimes become silent, with the development of occlusive calcification within the root canals. Even radiographically dark periapical areas have been known to disappear.

Epidermolysis bullosa

This inherited group of diseases is characterised by extreme fragility of the dermal and oral epithelium. An 'acquired' form, epidermolysis bullosa acquisita, is occasionally seen in association with *Crohn's disease*. Bulla formation and oral erosions may occur, which heal with gross scars, leading to limitation of movement of the lips, tongue and cheeks. Oral lesions may be precipitated by minor trauma, including that associated with mechanical dentistry. *Calendula* and *Arnica* should be employed regularly in the treatment of such cases. The prescription of remedies to inhibit or reduce excessive *scar tissue* formation should also be considered.

See also *Ulcers*.

Epistaxis, acute

This may occur as a result of the exacerbation of *blood pressure* in hypertensive patients who suffer from acute dental *anxiety*. It may also occur in non-hypertensives. Normal first-aid measures must be instituted. Both groups should be given *Ferrum phosphoricum* 30 every 15 minutes. Additionally and concurrently, the hypertensive should be given *Aconite* 30 every 15 minutes.

Epulis

The main types of epulis are the congenital epulis, the fibrous epulis and the giant cell epulis. Fibrous epulides occur much more commonly in women as opposed to men (4:1), and some are associated with pregnancy ('pregnancy epulis'). Giant cell epulides are rarely seen in adult males, and occur most commonly in children of either sex and women of fertile age. The pyogenic granuloma is a variant of the fibrous epulis in which the granulation tissue remains immature and vascular. Various homoeopathic internal remedies have been suggested for the treatment of epulides, including *Thuja, Calcarea carbonica, Natrum muriaticum,* Plumbum aceticum (lead acetate) and Lac caninum (bitch's milk). However, this is only of academic interest, since all these lesions should be removed surgically, with the normal homoeopathic precautions being taken as with *oral surgery* in general. Nevertheless, as a rule, Thuja 6 twice daily should be given after, perhaps for several months, in order to dissuade recurrence; although Natrum muriaticum 6 twice daily may be preferable in cases of pregnancy epulis.

Eruption, delayed dental

The principal remedies here are *Calcarea carbonica, Calcarea phosphorica,*
Silicea and *Calcarea fluorica*, given individually and according to susceptible typology, 6–12c twice daily. Difficult cases may additionally require
infrequent doses of *Bacillinum*. Other remedies, particularly *Sulphur* or
Fluoricum acidum, may occasionally be needed, based upon the constitutional aspects of the case.

   See also *Fluoridation*.

Eruption, disturbances associated with – *see* Teething

Erythema migrans – *see* Geographic tongue

Erythema multiforme

This inflammatory disease of sudden onset is usually self-limiting. The
symmetric skin lesions may be macular, papular, bullous, urticarial or
purpuric. So-called 'target' lesions with clear centres and erythematous
rings, or 'iris' lesions may occur. The skin lesions mainly present on the
extensor surfaces, but may be found on the palms or the soles. The oral
lesions consist of widespread and painful *ulceration* and blood-encrusted
lips. The disorder should be differentiated from primary herpetic *gingivo-*
stomatitis, the oral lesions of which may closely resemble those of
erythema multiforme. This may be difficult when the oral lesions are
manifest in the absence of those at other sites. The ocular and genital
mucosae may also be affected, and both lymphadenopathy and malaise
occur. More severe cases, with multiple site involvement, are termed
'Stevens-Johnson syndrome'. The attack generally resolves spontaneously in 7–14 days, but 2–3 recurrences of diminished severity may
occur over a period of 2–3 years following the initial manifestation of
the disease. Various causative factors are known, including: previous
infection with *Herpes simplex* virus or Mycoplasma pneumoniae, systemic
or topical drug therapies (especially sulphonamides and barbiturates),
pregnancy, exposure to sunlight, inflammatory bowel disease and allergy
to *foods* (especially benzoate-type preservatives).

   Local therapy may be given as for *aphthous ulcers*. Acquired infective
miasmatic cases may be given either Herpes simplex nosode 30–200
or Mycoplasma pneumoniae nosode 30, whichever is appropriate, in
infrequent dosages. Otherwise remedies may be given along the lines
suggested for primary herpetic *gingivostomatitis*. In persistent or
frequently recurrent cases, allergy to drugs, foods or preservatives may

be suspected. Thereafter, the administration of the offending drug or allergen in potency may be helpful (6–30c twice daily) or *Thuja* 6–30 twice daily may be considered.

Erythroplakia – *see* **Leukoplakia**

Espundia – *see* **Leishmaniasis, New World mucocutaneous**

Euphrasia (Euphrasia officinalis)
Homoeopathic eyebright. Both the diluted mother tincture and the potentised form are used in the treatment of acute *conjunctivitis*.

Evening primrose oil (EPO)
A good source of GLA (gamma-linolenic acid). Used as an adjunctive treatment in some female cases of *burning mouth syndrome*, recurrent *aphthous* ulceration, *atypical facial pain*, migraine and migrainous *neuralgia*. Also may be used in the treatment of neuropathy associated with *diabetes mellitus*. The usual adult dose is 500–1000mg (GLA 40–80mg) twice daily after food. Other sources of GLA, especially for those who cannot tolerate evening primrose oil (headaches, etc.) are borage oil, blackcurrant seed oil and starflower oil. GLA should not be used in cases of epilepsy (particularly temporal lobe epilepsy), breast cancer or mania. The role of GLA in preventing menopausal or postmenopausal alveolar ridge or periodontal bone loss is uncertain.

See also *Calcium; Periodontitis, chronic*.

Exfoliative cheilitis
This condition, restricted to the vermilion borders of the lips (predominantly the lower), is due to excessive production of keratin. Its aetiology is unknown. A similar condition, known as actinic cheilitis, results from exposure to sunlight. The regular use of *Calendula* ointment or cream may be helpful.

Exostosis – *see* **Fluoridation; Osteoma**

Exposure, pulpal – *see* **Pulpitis; Traumatised tooth**

Extraction – *see* **Oral surgery, prevention of complications in; Oral surgery, pain control after; Dry socket; Haemorrhage, acute dental; Sequestrum**

Fig. 18. Evening primrose

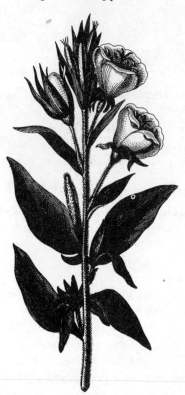

Extraction, botanic

I mention this peculiar subject out of interest. There are certain areas of the world where plant substances are inserted into the carious cavities of teeth in order to facilitate or promote extraction. In West Africa, the seed oil of Ximenia americana is employed for this purpose, as is the powdered root or bark of Acacia pennata soaked in palm wine. These are used to saturate cotton plugs, and appear to promote ease of extraction. The Panama Indians apparently insert the latex of either Hura crepitans or Chlorophora tinctoria into decayed teeth to induce spontaneous extraction. It is not possible to confirm either their safety or efficacy. The powdered dried root of the greater celandine (Chelidonium majus) was once used in England for similar purposes, but is essentially toxic.

Eye, 'something' in the – *see* Conjunctivitis, acute

Eye-strain

Consider *Ruta graveolens* 6–30 three times daily, and get your eyes checked.

F

Facial migraine – see Neuralgia, (periodic) migrainous

Facial nerve palsy (paralysis)

The two most commonly encountered types of facial nerve palsy are that associated with cerebrovascular accident (stroke, CVA) and *Bell's palsy.* Surgery or *tumours* of the parotid gland and non-surgical trauma are other causes. *Ramsay-Hunt syndrome* and *Lyme disease* should not be forgotten. Occasionally, facial nerve palsy is associated with intracranial tumours. In cases unassociated with surgery, a neurological opinion should be sought; some are a manifestation of *AIDS*. Facial palsy must be distinguished from other causes of facial weakness, such as myasthenia gravis. The remedy *Causticum* is one of prime importance in the treatment of lower motor neurone lesions of the facial nerve.

See also *Melkersson-Rosenthal syndrome.*

Facial pain (including oral & orofacial pain)

Apart from more obvious causes, such as *pulpitis, pericoronitis,* dental *abscess, fractures, salivary gland* disease, *tumours, Ramsay-Hunt syndrome* and sinusitis, there are a variety of diseases and syndromes in which facial, oral or orofacial pain is a dominant feature. These are considered under a number of different headings: *Burning mouth syndrome*; *Craniomandibular dysfunction* (TMJ dysfunction syndrome); *Facial pain, atypical* (which includes a discussion of atypical odontogenic pain); *Giant cell arteritis; Neuralgia, glossopharyngeal; Neuralgia, (periodic) migrainous* (which includes a discussion of migraine and paroxysmal facial hermicrania); *Neuralgia, post-herpetic; Neuralgia, trigeminal* (including pre-trigeminal neuralgia); *Paget's disease; Tension headache; TMJ, disorders of.*

Facial pain, atypical

This may be defined as a constant and virtually invariable dull ache of the face or jaw, present throughout the waking hours, lacking any obvious modalities, and with no obvious pathological cause. Atypical odontalgia is essentially the same disorder, but the pain is localised to one or more teeth.

This condition is more commonly experienced by women than men who, in general, are over the age of 30. Depression and early waking appear to be associated. Treatment with either the *Bach flower remedies* or major constitutional remedies, such as *Sepia* or *Natrum muriaticum* (according to the general and mental characteristics), is strongly indicated (in conjunction, perhaps, with *evening primrose oil)*. Indeed it is not unreasonable to consider this disorder as a psychologically determined variant of *craniomandibular dysfunction* (TMJ dysfunction syndrome). However, a small number of cases have diagnostically obscure physical origins. In some a non-vital but radiographically normal tooth is responsible. In others, *mercury toxicity* is the root of the matter.

Faint – *see* **Collapse, sudden**

Fear – *see* **Anxiety, acute dental**

Ferrum phosphoricum
Homoeopathic ferric phosphate. A remedy used in the treatment of acute *epistaxis, pulpitis*, the *traumatised tooth* with pulpitic symptoms and dental surgical *haemorrhage*. With regard to the latter, it is important to note the **susceptible typology:** weak, tired, pale and anaemic (especially children and adolescents).

Feverfew (Chrysanthemum/Pyrethrum parthenium)
Originally a botanic medicine, popularly used in the treatment of migraine, this has now been adopted by homoeopathy. The potentised remedy may be similarly used for migraine or migrainous *neuralgia*, and is effective in many *aphthous ulcer* cases. Its use for aphthous ulcers was suggested by the fact that a proportion of those taking crude feverfew developed painful ulceration of the oral mucosa.

Fibro-epithelial polyp
This is essentially scar tissue produced in response to repeated trauma, and is most commonly seen on the buccal mucosa in line with the occlusal plane. Rarely, other sites, such as the tongue, are involved. Correction of any malocclusion or recontouring of sharp teeth is indicated, together with surgical removal of the polyp, utilising the usual homoeopathic precautionary measures associated with *oral surgery* in general. Patients with a tendency to *keloid* formation may require other homoeopathic therapies.

Fibrous dysplasia

Of unknown aetiology, this condition is essentially the replacement of normal bone by fibrous tissue. In the monostotic type, a single bone is affected. With regard to the jaws, the maxilla is more commonly affected than the mandible, and there is a slowly developing unilateral and painless swelling during childhood. Alkaline phosphatase levels are normal. In the polyostotic type (many bones involved), about 20% of cases have jaw lesions, and the alkaline phosphatase level is raised. Approximately 50% of polyostotic cases exhibit hyperpigmentation of the skin. Albright's syndrome' is the term given to the combination of polyostotic fibrous dysplasia, skin hyperpigmentation and precocious female puberty.

The features of fibrous dysplasia, taken as a whole, strongly point to the remedies *Hekla lava*, *Calcarea fluorica* and *Calcarea phosphorica*. Their administration for a prolonged period during childhood may modify the progress of the disease. Calcarea phosphorica is well-indicated in Albright's syndrome. A sample prescription for the monostotic form might be: Hekla lava 6 twice daily plus Calcarea fluorica 12 at midday. For Albright's syndrome: Calcarea phosphorica 12 twice daily. Corrective *oral surgery* (with the usual homoeopathic precautions) may be required after the childhood growth phase.

Fibrous epulis – see Epulis

Fissure of lip – see Lip, median fissure of lower; Angular cheilitis

Fistula, oroantral

The principal remedy is *Silicea* 6 two or three times daily. Should this fail, give *Fluoricum acidum* 6 two or three times daily. Silicea is actually better indicated in overtly chilly individuals, and Fluoricum acidum in those who are hot.

Fluoricum acidum (Acidum fluoricum)

Homoeopathic fluoric acid. An important remedy for oroantral *fistula*, especially in hot individuals (generally < heat). Also used in the treatment of *osteomyelitis* and delayed *eruption*. **Susceptible typology:** hot, hair dull and dry, nails grow poorly and break easily, prone to varicose veins and ulcers, rough skin, pruritis of vulva or anus, pruritis around ulcers and fistular orifices.

Fluoridation

Despite the apparent past success of the fluoridation of water, topically applied fluoride and fluoride toothpastes, there is now a world-wide increase in caries in the 5 year-old group of developed countries. It seems likely that the same will be found in 12 year-olds. As it transpires, the apparent beneficial effects of fluoride, as determined statistically, are more likely accounted for by its ability to delay *eruption*. Hence, the importance of considering homoeopathy, once again, in the prevention of dental *caries*.

There are, of course, other problems with the mass fluoridation of water. Certain individuals, especially children, are excessively thirsty; in particular the *Phosphorus, Arsenicum album* and *Natrum muriaticum* types. They are, therefore, more prone to develop mottling and more serious manifestations of *fluorosis*. Moreover, individuals who have the susceptible typology of *Calcarea fluorica* are more sensitive to the adverse effects of fluoride. The adverse effects of fluoride are opposed by maintaining a high *calcium* intake (dairy products, canned fish, etc.).

There is a strong case for omitting fluoride from the composition of *toothpastes* for both adults and children.

Fluorosis

A disorder which, in its minor form, is only expressed as hypoplasia and mottling of the enamel of the teeth. In its intermediate form, multiple exostoses are produced. In its worst form, there is a crippling osteosclerosis. Fluorosis may also manifest as an increased susceptibility to traumatic *fracture*. It appears that, whilst the cancellous bone is increased in density, the cortex becomes thinner and more brittle.

Another study suggests the relationship between *fluoridation* of water supplies and osteosarcomata in males. It may indeed be responsible for increasing the incidence of other malignant *tumours*. It has also been suggested that the immune system is compromised by even small amounts of fluoride. Whether tiny amounts of fluoride have any essential function in man is uncertain.

Focal epithelial hyperplasia (Heck's disease)

This relatively rare disease dominantly affects Eskimos and North American Indians. It is characterised by numerous papillomatous lesions of the oral mucosa, which possibly are caused by human *papillomavirus* infection. Treatment with *Thuja* 6–12 twice daily may be helpful.

Focal sepsis

This is the concept that a silent periapical or parodontal infection may cause pathological effects at distant sites of the body. With regard to *subacute bacterial endocarditis*, this concept is recognised, but its application to other diseases is often denied. I know personally of only two such cases. One was a middle-aged male who developed a florid and widespread inflammatory arthritis, which subsequently responded to root canal filling and apicectomy of two non-vital lower incisors. The other was a gentleman of good repute, whose urethral discharge of non-venereal origin responded to the extraction of a non-vital premolar. The test for focal sepsis is to give the prime remedy for the chronic periapical or parodontal abscess, viz. *Hepar sulph.* 6 three times daily. Should there be significant improvement in the patient's condition, the presence of a silent area of periapical or parodontal infection is to be suspected and avidly sought.

Folate

Folate deficiency may be due to, amongst others, inadequate intake, *coeliac disease, tropical sprue*, and phenytoin or methotrexate therapy. It is not uncommon in pregnancy, and as a result of the use of the *contraceptive* pill or *hormone replacement therapy* (HRT). There may be *anaemia, burning mouth syndrome, angular cheilitis* and aphthous ulcers. The most marked oral manifestation is usually *glossitis*, the tongue becoming smooth (depapillated), red, shiny and painful. This appearance of the tongue is very similar to that of *vitamin B12* deficiency.

Replacement therapy (an adult dose of at least 5mg of folic acid daily by mouth) must not be given without proper analysis, advice or investigation. In epileptics taking phenytoin, exacerbation of the epilepsy may occur. There are also some tumours which are folate-dependent. If vitamin B12 deficiency is also present, then subacute combined degeneration of the spinal cord may be precipitated by giving folic acid alone.

Since folate deficiency may contribute to the development of *gingivitis* in those taking phenytoin, methotrexate, oral contraceptives or HRT, and those who are pregnant, some improvement may be secured by the use of folic acid *mouthwashes*. Gingivitis may be the only sign of mild folate deficiency, which is probably the most common deficiency state in the world.

Food allergy (including additive allergy)

In the dental field, this matter is of relevance to: *aphthous ulcers, burning mouth syndrome, dermatitis herpetiformis, lichenoid reactions, orofacial granulomatosis* and migrainous *neuralgia*. Food allergy may also be important in some cases of *tension headache* and migraine.

Fordyce's spots

These are normal structures, being sebaceous glands of the oral mucosa, varying considerably in number and distribution between individuals. They become more prominent during fevers, and are sometimes mistaken for pathological entities.

Foreign body

The expulsion of foreign bodies, such as buried silk sutures, amalgam and glass fragments, is encouraged by giving *Silicea* 6 three times daily. Where the foreign body is deeply situated (e.g. a broken needle fragment after an inferior dental nerve block), Silicea should not be given; for it is impossible to determine which way the foreign body might move. What many fail to realise is that Silicea only promotes the movement of a foreign body if there is a definite inflammatory reaction around it. A piece of shrapnel buried for years, with no tissue reaction of any significance, will not be caused to move; nor will a satisfactory prosthesis anywhere in the body. Only a dental *implant* already undergoing rejection will be extruded by Silicea.

Fracture, jaw

The most significant remedy for the promotion of union is *Symphytum* 6 three times daily, and this should be routinely given. The same remedy is usually of brilliant application in cases of non-union. At the same time, assessment of the general nutritional status of the patient is warranted. According to the case, *calcium* supplementation, *vitamin C* or *zinc* may be required. In the case of compound fractures, hot formentations of diluted *Calendula* Ø should be applied to the broken skin or oral mucosa. Calendula cream or ointment should be freely applied to the oral mucosa and lips after wiring.

In addition to Symphytum and Calendula, it may be necessary to administer other remedies concurrently. To relieve the pain of fractured bones, give *Rhus toxicodendron* 30 and *Bryonia* 30 in 2-hourly alternation. To relieve pain, when the bones are severely contused, give *Ruta* 30–200 2-hourly. For bruising of the soft tissues, use *Arnica* 30–200 three times daily. To promote sleep after injury, give Arnica as before, plus *Sticta pulmonaria* 200 two or three times daily. Where nerves have been damaged, give *Hypericum* 6–30 three times daily (for sensory nerves) or *Causticum* 6–30 three times daily (for motor nerves). Where non-union is persistent, despite the use of Symphytum and nutritional correction, consider Ruta 6–30 three times daily. For stiffness in the mobilising phase, consider Ruta 6–30 and Rhus toxicodendron 30 in 4-hourly alternation.

See also *Anaesthesia, general; Concussion; Fluorosis; Haematoma.*

Fragaria

Homoeopathic wood strawberry. In potency, Fragaria discourages the formation of dental calculus, causes existing calculus to soften (so that it may more readily be removed by *scaling*), and may even induce its 'spontaneous' disappearance. It is thus a useful adjunct in the treatment of *periodontitis* and *gingivitis*. There is no known susceptible typology in which Fragaria is particularly active in this respect, although the presence of a 'strawberry' *tongue* is believed to firmly indicate that it is appropriate.

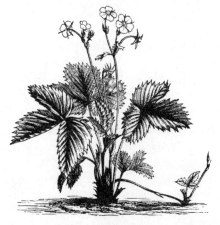

Fig. 19. Fragaria

Frey's syndrome (Auriculo-temporal syndrome)

This neurological condition may follow TMJ surgery, parotid surgery and injuries and injections in the same area. Frey's syndrome is sweating, and sometimes flushing, of the skin over the distribution of the auriculo-temporal nerve, produced by a stimulus to salivary secretion. It is thought to arise from the incorrect reconnection of nerve fibres following trauma, and appears about 5 weeks after the traumatic episode. Congential cases sometimes occur, probably as a result of birth trauma. Seldom is the condition sufficiently severe to warrant any treatment, but the avoidance of acid fruits or fruit juices may be helpful.

Frictional keratosis – *see* Keratosis, frictional

Fright – *see* Anxiety, acute dental

Fungal diseases

The most common fungal infection which affects the orofacial region is *candidosis*. Other rare forms of fungal infection are histoplasmosis, mucormycosis (predisposed to by diabetic acidosis, steriods and cytotoxic drugs), blastomycosis (North American blastomycosis) and paracoccidiomycosis (South American blastomycosis), for which the homoeopathic treatment is complex, and includes nosodes of the relevant organisms.

G

Gelsemium (Gelsemium sempervirens)*

Homoeopathic yellow jasmine. A remedy for the treatment of acute dental *anxiety*, where the patient is silent, motionless and exhibits a tremor. Diarrhoea sometimes accompanies these symptoms. A remedy for *migraine* and *tension headaches*. An important constitutional remedy. **Susceptible typology:** emotional, jumpy, fearful, thirstless, weak, trembles, prone to diarrhoea and 'paralysis' when anticipating an unpleasant event, < bad news, < heat or warmth, > sweating, > passing large quantities of urine, prone to migraine or tension headaches (beginning in the occiput, and radiating to the neck and shoulders).

Geographic tongue(Erythema migrans/Benign migratory glossitis)

This condition, which involves the dorsum and lateral aspects of the tongue, consists of irregular erythematous depapillated areas surrounded by pale margins of demarcation. These lesions improve and reappear at new sites, sometimes over the course of days, thus appearing to wander or migrate over the surface of the tongue. Even children may be affected. Some cases are associated with psoriasis. The majority of cases are

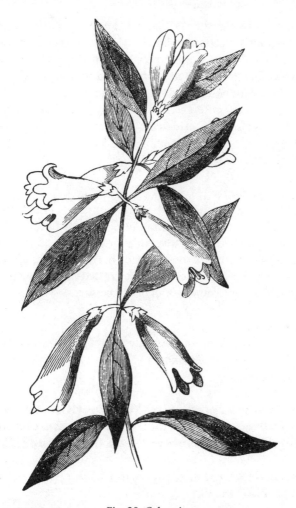

Fig. 20. Gelsemium

asymptomatic, but a few complain of soreness, especially with spicy food. Treatment is with *zinc* supplementation (adult dose: elemental zinc 15–30mg daily), together with *Taraxacum* 6–30 twice daily. Should these measures fail, consider *Natrum muriaticum* 6–12 twice daily. *Kali bichromicum* 6–30 twice daily also requires consideration.

Giant cell arteritis (Temporal arteritis)
This condition may affect vessels other than the temporal artery. Granulomatous lesions occur sporadically along the course of the artery.

Severe facial pain is often brought on by eating. Unlike most facial pain syndromes, it may be accompanied by weight loss, general muscle weakness and lethargy. The patient is typically over 60 years of age, and more likely a female. Since this condition may lead to blindness, early recognition and referral are essential,. Although initial treatment with *corticosteroids* is justified to preserve the vision, professional homoeopathic treatment should also be considered as part of the overall therapy.

Giant cell epulis – see Epulis

Giant cell granuloma
A giant cell lesion of the bone, which may produce extensive destruction. Its superficial presentation may be similar to that of a giant cell *epulis*. It is best removed surgically, with the normal homoeopathic precautions associated with *oral surgery*. Some of these lesions are associated with *hyperparathyroidism*, which must be treated appropriately. In such cases, oral surgical removal is usually unnecessary.

Gigantism, pituitary
The teeth in this condition are usually normal in size, but premature *eruption* of the permanent dentition and spacing are characteristic. *Hypercementosis* also develops.

Gingivitis, common chronic – see Periodontitis, chronic; *and also* Crohn's disease; Leukaemia; Orofacial granulomatosis; Pemphigoid, mucous membrane; von Willebrand's disease

Gingivitis, acute necrotising ulcerative (ANUG/Vincent's stomatitis/Trench mouth)
Local measures are important in the treatment of this acute bacterial disease, characterised by severe erosion of the gingival margins, loss of interdental papillae and extreme *halitosis*. The use of diluted hydrogen peroxide is of questionable benefit. Perhaps more important is the regular use (three or four times daily) of *Propolis* mouthwashes, combined with the application of undiluted Propolis Ø to the gingival margins and interdental spaces once or twice daily, and thorough dental hygiene. Internally, homoeopathic therapy may be of immense benefit. The key remedy is undoubtedly *Mercurius solubilis* 30 three times daily, especially where the tongue is heavily coated. Where the tongue is clean, *Nitricum acidum* 30 three times daily is better indicated. Where improvement is

slow under the influence of the former remedies and there has been much destruction of gingival tissue, consider *Kali chloricum* 30 three times daily. Some cases of *glandular fever* are associated with a gingivitis similar to that of *ANUG*, and these may require additional treatment with Glandular fever nosode 30.

See also *Pellagra.*

Gingivitis, phenytoin

The use of phenytoin in epilepsy may lead to hyperplastic gingivitis. Correct oral hygiene is essential, together with the use of 0.1% folic acid *mouthwashes* twice daily. The mouthwash must not be swallowed. *Thuja* 6–12 twice daily may be helpful.

See also *Folate.*

Gingivitis, pregnancy

Hormonal changes in pregnancy increase the likelihood of gingivitis. 'Pregnancy *epulis*' may also arise. Strict oral hygiene and the regular use of *Myrrh* mouthwashes are strongly indicated. Homoeopathic remedies should be prescribed on the basis of the constitution acquired in pregnancy and not that which preceded it. Remedies to be particularly considered are *Natrum muriaticum* and *Sepia*. These, or others selected, should not be given in too high a potency. *Coenzyme Q10* should not be administered in pregnancy, but folic acid 400mcg–5mg daily and *zinc* (15mg elemental zinc daily) may be used routinely as an adjunctive therapy. The use of 0.1% folic acid *mouthwashes* twice daily is recommended in addition to those of Myrrh.

See also *Folate.*

Gingivitis, puberty

Hormonal changes, particularly in girls, at puberty may favour the development of gingivitis. Good oral hygiene, *Myrrh* mouthwashes, *coenzyme Q10* (30mg daily) and *zinc* (elemental zinc 15–30mg daily) may all be helpful. Homoeopathic remedies prescribed on a constitutional basis are also of service; in particular, *Calcarea phosphorica, Ignatia, Natrum muriaticum, Pulsatilla* and *Sepia*, according to susceptible typology. In severely depressed cases with overt *halitosis, Aurum metallicum* 30 and higher twice daily should be considered, but since some may be suicidal, expert advice should be sought before prescribing.

Gingivostomatitis, primary herpetic

The majority of cases occur in childhood. It is less commonly seen in adults, in whom the disease is generally of greater severity. Some cases in children may be confused with the oral manifestations of acute *leukaemia* and a blood test may be required for differentiation (some diagnostic confusion may also arise with respect to *erythema multiforme*). This vesicular, and subsequently ulcerative, condition may affect the lips as well as the oral mucosa (compare *herpangina*). Local treatment includes *Calendula* or *Propolis* mouthwashes, creams or ointments. The topical application of *vitamin E* is said to produce effective pain relief within 15 minutes; this may be applied either directly or as an ointment. Internally, a key remedy is *Mercurius solubilis* 6–30 three times daily, especially if there is much salivation. With a dry mouth, prostration and drowsiness, *Baptisia* 30 three times daily is better indicated. Occasionally, in severe cases, concurrent treatment with *Herpes simplex* nosode 30 once daily will be required.

Glandular fever (Infectious mononucleosis)

Approximately 30% of glandular fever cases exhibit purpura or petechiae in the palate and pseudomembranous oral *ulceration*. Unilateral *pericoronitis* or a condition of the gingivae resembling *ANUG* may also occur. Local treatments are similar to those for *aphthous ulcers*, common pericoronitis and ANUG. Internal treatment includes the use of Glandular fever nosode 30.

See also *Thrombocytopenia; Zinc.*

Glossitis

This may occur as a result of *iron, folate, vitamin B12, vitamin B2* or niacin deficiency.

See also *Candidosis, oral; Geographic tongue* (Benign migratory glossitis); *Median rhomboid glossitis* (Superficial midline glossitis); *Pellagra.*

Glossodynia

Another term for *burning mouth syndrome*, where the tongue is affected.

Glossopharyngeal neuralgia – *see* Neuralgia, glossopharyngeal

Glossopyrosis

Another term for *burning mouth syndrome*, where the tongue is affected.

Gonorrhoea

Orogenital contact may result in the transmission of this disease to the mouth. The patient complains of a painful oral mucosa, *halitosis* and perversion of *taste*. Clinical signs include: lymphadenopathy, erythema, oedema, *ulceration* and pseudomembrane formation (particularly in the oropharynx). Referral is essential.

Gout

Gout is common, but rare in the TMJ. Its principal relevance to dentistry, however, is that some cases may be associated with *hypercementosis*.

Granatum

Homoeopathic pomegranate root bark. A remedy for painful cracking of the *TMJ* and *sialorrhoea*. **Susceptible typology:** hungry, thin or emaciated, prone to digestive upsets and itching (especially of palms).

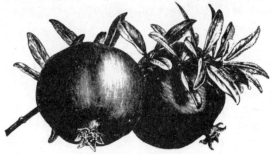

Fig. 21. Granatum

Granulocytopenia – *see* Agranulocytosis

Granuloma inguinale

This is essentially a venereal bacterial disease of the tropics and sub-tropics, but may be seen occasionally elsewhere. A papule develops, which *ulcerates* to produce a mass of granulations. Occasionally, the mouth is involved, with subsequent formation of excessive *scar tissue*, and limitation of opening.

Graphites*

Homeopathic pencil-lead. A remedy for *keloid* scar formation, and a major consitutional remedy. **Susceptible typology:** fat, chilly (but > walking in fresh air), dyspeptic, anaemic, constipated, sad, weepy (< music). Many Graphites subjects are menopausal.

Grinspan's syndrome

The term applied to the combination of *diabetes mellitus*, high *blood pressure* and oral *lichenoid reaction*. The lichenoid component of the triad is probably due to the antihypertensive or oral hypoglycaemic drugs used in treatment.

Gum-boil – *see* Abscess, dental

Gunpowder

Homoeopathic black gunpowder. A remedy for boils and *incisional abscess*.

Gustatory sweating & flushing

This is a normal bilateral phenomenon after the ingestion of chili, pepper or ginger. However, when it occurs unilaterally and in relation to many foods, it is usually a manifestation of *Frey's syndrome*.

H

Haemangioma (Vascular naevus)

Most haemangiomata of the orofacial region are congenital malformations of the blood vessels. Capillary and cavernous types are described. Long-term treatment with *Calcarea fluorica* 6–12 twice daily may be helpful in some cases to reduce their size. *Haemorrhage* from trauma may be controlled with *Arnica* and hot formentations of *Calendula*.

See also *Kaposi's sarcoma*.

Haematoma

This may be treated with *Arnica* 30–200 three times daily. If the haematoma is extraoral, then Arnica Ø may be applied several times daily, but only to unbroken skin.

Haemophilia

Classical haemophilia (haemophilia A) is associated with factor VIII deficiency. Christmas disease (haemophilia B) is associated with factor IX deficiency. They are clinically similar. The dental surgeon must not expect *Arnica* and other remedies for dental *haemorrhage* to substitute for replacement of the missing factors. However, the combination of replacement and homoeopathic therapy may be fruitful in many cases.

Haemorrhage, acute dental

Excessive haemorrhage from extraction or surgery in general is usually preventable by giving *Arnica* 30–200 three times daily for one day prior to the procedure, with an extra dose immediately before. After the procedure, the same remedy may be given as often as once every 15–30 minutes to control haemorrhage, and thereafter three times daily for about 7 days. *Hypericum* 30 is often given along with Arnica, three times daily, to control pain and promote the repair of sensory nerves. Hot fomentations of *Calendula* are also of service in the control of surgical haemorrhage. Haematoma formation following *local anaesthesia* is also preventable and treatable with Arnica.

Occasionally, however, surgical haemorrhage is not controlled by satisfactory suturing and the homoeopathic measures discussed previously. Other remedies will be required. *Phosphorus* 30–200 is undoubtedly the key remedy in many cases of bright red bleeding, but sometimes fails. With persistent bright red bleeding, a useful mixture is *China* 6 + Phosphorus 12 + *Ferrum phosphoricum* 30. Should this fail, consider *Ipecacuanha* 30 + *Millefolium* 30. These mixtures should be premixed in liquid potency, in order that they may be swiftly administered. In cases of persistent dark bleeding, *Lachesis* 30 is better indicated. Any of the former remedies should be given every 10 minutes, until the haemorrhage is arrested. Thereafter, proceed with Arnica three times daily.

Repeated episodes of prolonged or excessive bleeding associated with *oral surgery* suggest the presence of an haemorrhagic disease, which may be due to the lack of certain clotting factors, platelet deficiency, Warfarin therapy or defects of the capillaries. Special precautions and therapies will be required (such as the replacement of clotting factors), which are outside the scope of the average dental practice. Referral to specialist centres is warranted. Some cases may be merely associated with *vitamin C* deficiency from an inadequate diet.

See also *Ehlers-Danlos syndrome; Haemophilia; Hereditary haemorrhagic telangiectasia; Leukaemia; Thrombocytopenia; von Willebrand's disease.*

Hairy leukoplakia – *see* AIDS; Leukoplakia

Hairy tongue – *see* Tongue, black hairy

Halitosis (Offensive or foul breath)

This is often due to poor oral hygiene, the excessive use of tobacco, the consumption of pungent foods, or the presence of oral disease, such as chronic *periodontitis*. Appropriate rectification of these problems will eliminate halitosis. However, in some instances, halitosis is not of oral origin, but stems from a disease of the throat, sinuses or stomach, which, in turn, may be part of a general constitutional problem. In some cases, the excretion of noxious substances in the breath is the body's attempt to remove accumulated toxins; diabetic ketosis being an extreme example. Halitosis appears temporarily with detoxifying diets, such as grape cures, juice fasts and elimination diets for food allergy.

Apart from the treatment of periodontal disease itself, remedies may be usefully employed in the treatment of halitosis of non-dental origin. The principal remedies to be considered in this respect are *Arsenicum album*, *Aurum metallicum*, *Chamomilla*, *Graphites*, *Kali phosphoricum*, *Kreasotum*, *Lachesis*, *Mercurius solubilis*, *Natrum muriaticum*, *Nitricum acidum*, *Nux vomica*, *Phytolacca*, *Pulsatilla*, *Spigelia* and *Sulphur*. A prescription based upon the susceptible typology will generally be better than one dominantly selected on the basis of the character of the halitosis (that is to say, the nature of the smell and its modalities, e.g. < after eating).

One particular case of mine is of special interest. This was a child with a fishy breath who failed to respond to normally well-indicated remedies. The root of the problem turned out to be a diptheria-pertussis-tetanus immunisation. The miasmic hangover was eliminated by a few intermittent doses of the nosode of the vaccine, whereupon the halitosis disappeared.

See also *Gonorrhoea*.

Hand, foot & mouth disease

This *Coxsackievirus* (A4, A5, A9, A10, A16) disease often occurs in epidemic form. Vesicular eruptions occur on the hands, feet, pharyngeal mucosa, buccal sulcus, tongue and soft palate. The cutaneous lesions resolve within 3 days, there is little systemic disturbance, and the whole disease clears spontaneously in 7–10 days. Local oral treatment with *Calendula* or *Myrrh* mouthwashes is the principal therapy.

See also *Ulcers*.

Headache – *see* Facial pain

Heck's disease – *see* Focal epithelial hyperplasia

Hekla lava

Homoeopathic preparation of the finer volcanic ash from Mount Hekla,

Iceland (formerly believed to be the gateway to Hell). A remedy with important actions on the bones of the jaws. Used in the treatment of *dry socket, exostoses,* expansive *tumours and cysts* of the jaws (including periapical cysts), *fibrous dysplasia* (especially of the maxilla). *Paget's disease* and *osteomyelitis.* The modality of the lesion '< touch and pressure', encourages its selection, but is not essential for all cases. Amongst other constituents, Hekla lava contains silica and lime. The **susceptible typology** for its full action is thus related to those of *Silicea* and the *Calcareae* (particularly *Calcarea fluorica* and *Calcarea phosphorica*). Compare *Lapis albus.*

See also *Endodontics.*

Hemicrania, paroxysmal facial – see **Neuralgia, (periodic) migrainous**

Hepar sulph. (Hepar sulphuris calcareum Hahnemannii) *

Homoeopathic impure calcium sulphide (prepared by burning the white interior of oyster shells with pure flowers of sulphur in a crucible). The most important general remedy for dental *abscess* and *periocoronitis,* irrespective of susceptible typology (although swifter in action in those of the appropriate typology). Lower potencies, such as 6c, encourage suppuration. Higher potencies, such as 30c, stop or cause the reabsorption of pus (see *Endodontics*). Hepar sulph. 30–200 may be given in cases of *pulpitis,* but lower potencies should never be given to treat this condition. **Susceptible typology:** flabby, chilly (< dry cold and cold draughts), indolent, irritable, easily angered, unhealthy skin, skin sensitive to touch, prone to catching infections, children have lymphadenopathy (very sensitive to touch).

Hereditary haemorrhagic telangiectasia (Rendu-Osler-Weber disease)

This inherited disorder is characterised by the appearance of numerous haemangiomatous or telangiectatic lesions of the oral mucosa and skin. These bleed readily with trauma. Special care is thus required during all dental procedures. *Arnica* should be used routinely, and hot *Calendula* formentations should be at hand. *Calcarea fluorica* 6–12 twice daily may reduce the risk of haemorrhage.

Herpangina

This relatively mild disease, due to various *Coxsackieviruses* (A2, A4–A6,

A8) occurs mainly in children. Multiple small vesicles appear on the oral mucosa (particularly on the soft palate) and the oropharynx, which subsequently *ulcerate*. The distribution within the oral cavity is dominantly posterior (compare primary herpetic *gingivostomatitis*). Fever may also occur. *Propolis, Myrrh* or *Calendula* mouthwashes or gargles may be helpful, together with *Mercurius solubilis* 6–12 three times daily.

Herpes labialis (Cold sore)

This is the more common orofacial manifestation of secondary herpes simplex infection, resulting from reactivation of the dormant virus. Such factors as fatigue, sun, infections, and menstruation may precipitate its onset. A good local application for cold-sores, which lessens the pain and duration, is prepared by mixing 10 drops of *Propolis* Ø and 10 drops of *tea tree oil* with 50g of aqueous cream. This should be applied 3–6 times daily, and is useful in many cases. Internally, *Natrum muriaticum* 30 three times daily is probably the most successful remedy, especially in hot people. In chilly individuals (and especially in women), *Sepia* 6–12 three times daily is better indicated. Should these measures fail, consider *Rhus toxicodendron* 30 three times daily or Herpes simplex nosode 30 twice daily. Supplementary therapy with *vitamin C* 600mg plus mixed *bioflavonoids* 600mg three times daily may also promote healing.

For the treatment of the predisposition to cold sores, constitutional therapy is indicated according to the susceptible typology. The key remedies to be considered are Natrum muriaticum, Sepia and *Sulphur*. Long-term *zinc* (15–30mg daily) and vitamin C (1–2g daily) supplementation may also be helpful. There may be an association in some cases between recurrent herpes labialis and *iron* deficiency. Injections of *vitamin B12* 1000mcg, initially every two weeks may be helpful in some cases.

The less common orofacial manifestation of secondary herpes simplex infection is the occurrence of ulceration of the oral mucosa. The sites most frequently involved are the attached gingivae, the hard palate and the buccal mucosa. In such cases, the local treatment is similar to that for primary herpetic *gingivostomatitis,* and the systemic treatment follows the lines given above for herpes labialis. Intraoral or perioral secondary herpes simplex lesions can be associated with *AIDS*.

See also *Aphthous ulcers* (for L-lysine therapy); Syphilis (with regard to chancre).

Herpes simplex infection – *see* AIDS; Erythema multiforme; Gingivostomatitis, primary herpetic; Herpes labialis. *See also under* **Aphthous ulcers** *for L-lysine therapy*

Herpes zoster (Shingles)
This condition, which is the reactivation of a dormant chickenpox (Varicella zoster) virus, may affect one side of the face, and is generally amenable to homoeopathic treatment. The key remedy is *Rhus toxicodendron* 12–30 three times daily, which will often shorten the duration of the disorder. Ophthalmic herpes zoster, however, is usually better treated with *Prunus spinosa* 12–30 three to four times daily. Varicella nosode 30 may also be given concurrently, once daily. A Rhus toxicodendron cream (Rhus toxicodendron Ø 20 drops in 50g of aqueous cream) may be applied to the skin (neither near the eye nor in the mouth), 3–6 times daily. Intramuscular or deep subcutaneous injections of *vitamin* B12 500mcg daily appear to produce pain relief and rapid healing. Intravenous *vitamin* C is also believed to be helpful.

Kali phosphoricum is of great service in preventing and treating postherpetic neuralgia. Treatment may be complemented with *Vitamin E* 600IU daily by mouth and vitamin B12 by injection, 1000mcg daily for 6 days, followed by the same dose once weekly for 6 weeks.

See also *Neuralgia, post-herpetic; AIDS; Ramsay-Hunt syndrome.*

Histoplasmosis – *see* Fungal diseases

Hormone replacement therapy (HRT) – *see* Folate; Vitamin B6

Human papillomavirus – *see* Papillomavirus lesions, human

Hydrastis (Hydrastis canadensis)
Botanic and homoeopathic. Goldenseal. The mother tincture, prepared from the roots, is useful in the treatment of oral *candidosis* and is sometimes employed in the treatment of *aphthous ulcers*. A *mouthwash*, which should not be swallowed, is prepared by adding 30 drops of Ø to 250ml of water. The potentised remedy is also utilised in the treatment of aphthous ulcers. Viscid saliva and an imprinted *tongue*, especially in tired and thin individuals, indicates its suitability (compare *Kali bichromicum*).

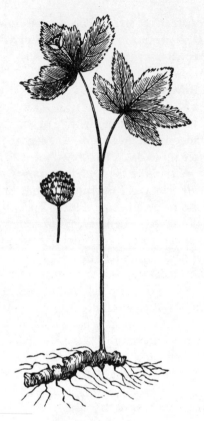

Fig. 22. Hydrastis

Hydroxocobalamin – see **Vitamin B12**

Hypercementosis
Abnormal thickening of the cementum may lead to difficulty in extraction. It is associated with pituitary *gigantism* and *Paget's disease*. Other cases are related to hyperthyroidism and *gout*. Some merely occur as a result of familial inheritance in the absence of any major coexistent disorders.

Hypericum (Hypericum perforatum)
Homoeopathic St. John's wort (see frontispiece). A remedy for injured *nerves* or nerve endings, and trauma to the cerebrospinal system, irrespective of susceptible typology. It is often prescribed (30c three times daily) concurrently with *Arnica*, the great remedy for *haemorrhage* in

dental surgery. It controls the pain of traumatised nerves. It promotes the regeneration of severed nerves, and has been described as 'the Arnica of the nervous system'. However, my own feeling is that it is primarily a remedy for sensory nerves, whereas *Causticum* is better indicated in trauma to motor nerves. It is also a remedy for post-herpetic and trigeminal *neuralgia*, where lancinating shooting pains occur, and there is aggravation by the least contact or movement. Its use has been suggested in cases of *craniomandibular dysfunction*, especially if *trismus* is present.

See also *Anaesthesia, local; Concussion; Oral surgery, pain control after; Pulpitis; Traumatised tooth.*

Hyperparathyroidism

This may be due to an adenoma of the parathyroid glands (primary hyperparathyroidism) or may be secondary to renal disease (secondary hyperparathyroidism). Radiographically, there is complete or partial loss of the lamina dura and a ground-glass appearance of the alveolus. The serum calcium and alkaline phosphatase levels are raised. In the jaws and elsewhere, giant cell lesions (see *Epulis*) and *cysts* may develop. Oral lesions generally resolve with satisfactory treatment of the underlying disorder.

Hyperpigmentation – *see* Pigmentation, oral & circumoral

Hyperpituitarism – *see* Acromegaly; Gigantism, pituitary

Hyperplastic gingivitis – *see* Gingivitis, phenytoin; Leukaemia

Hyperthyroidism

It is claimed that *hypercementosis* is commoner in those who suffer from this disorder.

Hypothyroidism

In the adult form of the disease, there is a puffy face with a sleepy appearance, and sometimes loss of the outer eyebrows. In the juvenile form (cretinism), there is macroglossia, enlargement of the lips, underdevelopment of the mandible and maxillary hypoplasia. Replacement therapy is invariably indicated, although some mild adult cases respond well to homoeopathic treatment, enabling them to reduce or eliminate their conventional medication.

See also *Thyropenia.*

I

Ignatia (Ignatia amara)*

Homoeopathic St. Ignatius' bean (Strychnos ignatia). A remedy for the treatment of certain psychological or psychosomatic states. It is employed in the treatment of acute dental *anxiety, bruxism and bruxomania, burning mouth syndrome, xerostomia, craniomandibular dysfunction, gingivitis* of puberty, migraine, migrainous *neuralgia* and *tension headache*. It may be prescribed in 6–200c two or three times daily according to sensitivity and response. It is only indicated by the appropriate **susceptible typology:** excessively sensitive to pain and stress of any kind, sighs frequently, changeable moods, cries easily but soon changes to laughter (and vice versa), forgets problems easily when distracted, spectacular hysterical behaviour, hypersensitive to smells (especially tobacco), sometimes a sensation of a lump in the throat (globus hystericus). The Ignatia patient is made worse generally by even small amounts of coffee. This Ignatia syndrome, as it might be termed, may be a basic constitutional state stemming from a severe emotional upset in the past (such as the loss of a loved one), or a transient state associated with temporary psychological trauma (such as a visit to the dentist).

Impetigo

A highly contagious bacterial infection of childhood, usually involving the facial skin. It is characterised by honey-coloured crusts overlying red areas of denuded skin. Infection may readily pass to the dental surgeon, his assistant, or, via instruments or linen, to other patients. Treatment involves the use of *Propolis* or *tea tree oil* cream (20 drops of Ø or oil in 50g aqueous cream) 3–6 times daily, and the initial use internally of *Antimonium crudum* 6–12 three times daily. Should this fail, consider *Mezereum* 6–30 three times daily.

Implants, dental

For some months after the insertion of an implant, the remedy *Silicea* should not be given, in that it may induce extrusion. Once an implant is successful and is not subject to rejection, this remedy may be given freely where it is indicated. *Arnica* should be administered both before and after the procedure. *Symphytum* 6 three times daily should be given in order to encourage bone formation around the implant.

Incisional abscess

This should be treated externally with hot *Calendula* formentations. Internally, *Gunpowder* 6 three times daily should be given initially. Once discharge of pus has occurred, switch to *Silicea* 6–12 three times daily.

Infection, prevention of, in oral surgery – *see* Pyrogen; Subacute endocarditis, prevention of

Infectious mononucleosis – *see* Glandular fever

Infective endocarditis – *see* Subacute bacterial endocarditis, prevention of

Inferior dental nerve injury – *see* Nerve injury

Influenza, prevention of – *see* Colds & influenza, prevention of

Iodum*

Homoeopathic iodine. An important constitutional remedy. **Susceptible typology:** anxious, depressed, introverted, ravenous appetite but remains thin, < heat, always seeking cool surroundings, prone to throbbing sensations, diarrhoea from milk, prone to hyperthyroidism, *tongue* indented.

Ipecacuanha

Homoeopathic preparation of the roots of Uragoga ipecacuanha (Brazil). A remedy for nausea following *general anaesthesia*, and dental *haemorrhage*. In dental haemorrhage, it is indicated by bright red bleeding, especially if accompanied by severe nausea and excessive salivation.

Iris versicolor

Homoeopathic blue flag iris. A remedy for migraine or migrainous *neuralgia*, irrespective of laterality, preceded by clouding of vision or fortification spectra. The characteristic pain is one of intense burning. Iris versicolour is also sometimes employed in the treatment of *burning mouth syndrome* in migrainous patients.

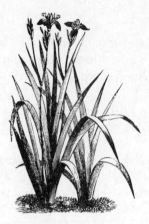

Fig. 23. Iris versicolor

Iron

Iron deficiency is most often caused by excessive loss or defective utilisation. The oral signs of iron deficiency anaemia are: atrophic *glossitis* (a smooth and sometimes pale tongue), general thinning of the oral mucosa, predisposition to *aphthous ulcers* and *angular cheilitis*. Kelly-Paterson (Plummer-Vinson) syndrome is the triad of iron deficiency anaemia, dysphagia and post-cricoid oesophageal stricture. It is associated with a higher risk of developing oral and postcricoid *carcinoma*. In all cases of iron deficiency, the cause should be established, and treated appropriately (heavy periods, etc.). Supplementary therapy is best given as a single dose of chelated iron 28mg daily, together with *vitamin C* 100mg administered at the same time (note that adult iron supplements can be very dangerous for small children). One important point concerning iron deficiency is that the body's iron stores may be severely depleted before overt changes occur in the red blood cells (microcytosis and reduced haemoglobin). Where the conjunctivae of the lower eyelids are pale, but the blood film is normal, it is important to proceed to a further blood test to assess the ferritin level. Oral manifestations may precede the onset of frank iron deficiency anaemia. There may be an association between iron deficiency and recurrent *herpes labialis* or *burning mouth syndrome*. Iron supplementation is contraindicated in cases of *thalassaemia minor*.

See also *Haemorrhage, acute dental; Tropical sprue*.

J

Jaborandi

Homoeopathic preparation of Pilocarpus jaborandi (Brazil), the principal alkaloid of which is pilocarpine. A remedy for *mumps* and *sialorrhoea*. A leading indication is the association of excessive salivation and excessive sweating.

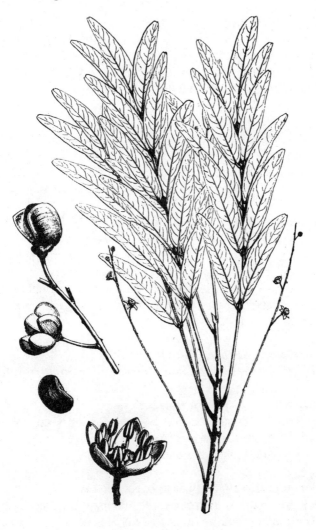

Fig. 24. Jaborandi

Jaw claudication

An inaccurate term used to describe the phenomenon of pain on eating associated with *giant cell arteritis*. The pain is not brought on by ischaemia, unlike intermittent claudication of the legs in cases of artherosclerosis.

K

Kali bichromicum (Kalium bichromicum)

Homoeopathic potassium bichromate. Used in the treatment of *aphthous ulcers*. It is particularly indicated where they have a yellow or yellow-green base, the *tongue* is imprinted, the mouth dry, the saliva viscid and the patient plump and catarrhal (compare *Hydrastis*). Other tongue signs indicative of the remedy are: red, shining, smooth, dry and *geographic tongue*. It is also indicated in *black hairy tongue, median rhomboid glossitis* and in the treatment of suborbital migrainous *neuralgia*, where the pain is distinctly localised, preceded by visual disturbance and > pressure. Kali bichromicum is most active in chilly and plump individuals. It is an important remedy in the treatment of sinusitis and *xerostomia*.

Kali carbonicum (Kalium carbonicum)*

Homoeopathic potassium carbonate. A remedy sometimes indicated in the treatment of chronic *gingivitis* and *periodontitis*. An important constitutional remedy. **Susceptible typology:** anxious, easily discouraged, sensitive to the least noise and pain, anxiety felt in the pit of the stomach, weary, anaemic, flabby, obese, sweaty, oedema of face or upper eyelids, < cold.

Kali chloricum (Kalium chloricum)

Homoeopathic potassium chlorate. A remedy for *cancrum oris* and *ANUG*.

Kali muriaticum (Kalium muriaticum)

Homoeopathic potassium chloride. A secondary remedy for oral *candidosis,* where *Borax* fails. It is especially indicated in patients who are < fatty or rich foods (including *Pulsatilla* types).

Kali phosphoricum (Kalium phosphoricum)

Homoeopathic potassium phosphate. Perhaps the best remedy for the prevention and treatment of post-herpetic *neuralgia*. Also useful in the treatment of *tension headaches* of students and *halitosis*. **Susceptible**

typology: tired, weak, hypersensitive, mentally exhausted (from mental work, sexual excesses, recurrent illnesses).

Kalmia latifolia

Homoeopathic mountain laurel. A remedy for severe facial *neuralgia*, involving the right eye and < movement. It is especially indicated in rheumatic subjects.

Kaposi's sarcoma

This is a malignant endothelial neoplasm, which appears as a bluish or purple patch on the palate. It is almost exclusively seen as a complication of *AIDS*.

See also *Tumours & cysts*.

Kelly-Paterson syndrome – see Iron

Keloid – see Scar tissue, excessive

Keratosis, frictional

White keratotic patches may arise from *prosthetic* or dental irritation. These should disappear once the source of irritation (e.g. a sharp tooth) has been corrected. Those that persist for more than three weeks after the apparent cause has been removed should be biopsied.

See also *Leukoplakia*.

Keratosis, smoker's

Smoker's keratosis usually appears as a diffuse whitening of any area of the oral mucosa that has repeatedly come in contact with smoke. In the palate, the mucous glands become enlarged and their orifices show as red dots. The condition will resolve with abstinence, perhaps assisted by *Calendula* mouthwashes. There is a higher incidence of oral *carcinoma* in smokers, the risk of which is possibly diminished by the regular administration of *vitamin E* 600IU daily.

Koplik's spots – see Measles

Krameria (Ratanhia)

Botanic. The root of Krameria triandra (Peruvian krameria), found in Bolivia and Peru, has useful properties in the topical treatment of *gingivitis* and *periodontitis*. It is incorporated into some botanic *toothpastes*.

Kreasotum

Homoeopathic creosote. A remedy for *halitosis*. It is useful for early and significant *caries* of the deciduous teeth, where it may reduce the predisposition. It is especially indicated in thin and weedy children. Its use may also be considered in adults with a predisposition to gross caries, where the gums are spongy and bleeding (*gingivitis*). They must hurry when a desire comes to urinate, the urine being offensive.

L

L-lysine therapy – *see* **Aphthous ulcers**

Lachesis *

Homoeopathic bushmaster (snake) venom. A remedy for dark dental *haemorrhage, burning mouth syndrome, ranula, halitosis* of non-dental origin and *xerostomia*. An important constitutional remedy, particularly of the menopause and in alcoholics. **Susceptible typology:** excessively loquacious, jealous, vindictive, proud, suspicious, disturbing dreams, prone to depression and sulking, hot with hot flushes, plethoric face, blotchy skin, intolerance of tight clothing, dislikes being touched or constricted, dry tongue, complaints mainly left-sided or move from left to right.

Lapis albus

Homoeopathic calcium silicofluoride. A remedy for enlargement of the cervical or *salivary glands, pleomorphic salivary adenoma* and *salivary calculus*. Firmness of the gland, together with a certain elasticity or pliability suggests the use of this remedy. Consistent with its chemical composition, it is especially indicated in persons of *Silicea* or *Calcarea fluorica* **typology**.

Laryngitis in dental surgeons

Either *Argentum metallicum* or *Arum triphyllum* is strongly indicated in the communicative, according to symptoms. Either may be given in a potency of 30c three times daily.

Latrodectus (Latrodectus mactans)

Homoeopathic preparation of the black widow spider. A useful emergency remedy for *angina pectoris*.

Ledum (Ledum palustre)

Homoeopathic marsh tea. A remedy for injuries from sharp instruments (puncture wounds), especially in those which have not bled significantly (otherwise, *Arnica* is more applicable). The site of puncture feels either cold to the patient or to the practitioner. Useful in the treatment of jaw stiffness following *local anaesthesia.*

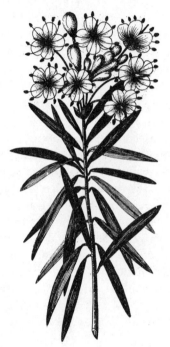

Fig. 25. Ledum

Leshmaniasis, New World mucocutaneous (Espundia)

This disease is caused by certain species of the protozoan parasite Leishmania, contracted via the bite of a sand-fly. It is found in certain areas of South and Central America, but can develop also in those who return home after a trip. There may be considerable destruction of the facial structures, resembling an advanced malignant *tumour* of the orofacial region, from which it must be differentiated. Homoeopathy may be helpful in treatment, including the use of a specific nosode.

Leukaemia

This disorder of leukocytes may occur in either acute or chronic forms, both of which have oral manifestations. Chronic leukaemia may be associated with oral *candidosis, ulceration, herpes simplex infection* and petechiae. Oral signs in acute leukaemia are severe and rapidly progressive. They are essentially the same as those for the chronic type, but more florid, with considerable gingival hypertrophy and gingival *haemorrhage*. Urgent referral is warranted. The dental surgeon may be the first to diagnose the disease.

Leukoplakia

This is defined as a white patch of the oral mucosa, which cannot be wiped away, and is not definable pathologically or clinically as any other orthodox disease entity. Erythroplakia is an associated erythematous patch, defined similarly. From the practical point of view, although many such lesions may be histologically benign, all should be regarded as having malignant potential, and frequent observation is thus required. Although the definition of leukoplakia successfully excludes *lichen planus* and most forms of oral *candidosis*, it is essential to place upon it a rider which includes candidal leukoplakia, which is a potentially malignant condition. Hairy leukoplakia is especially seen as a complication of *AIDS*.

Concerning natural therapy, apart from the correction of alcohol or tobacco habits, the paper by S.E. Benner et al (J. Nat. Cancer Inst., 85 (1), 44–47, 1993) is worthy of mention. It was shown that the administration of 400IU of *vitamin E* twice daily for 24 weeks caused regression of the condition in 46% of patients, with 31% of patients showing histological responses.

See also *Keratosis, frictional; Papillomavirus lesions, human; Syphilis.*

Lichen planus

This is a mucocutaneous disorder which affects up to 2% of the population of the UK, and is more prevalent in women.

Characteristically, violaceous flat-topped papules appear on the flexor surfaces of the wrists. The intraoral appearance is variable, and the disease may affect any site. It is essentially a benign condition, and when it appears as white patches, it must be differentiated from *leukoplakia*. Various types are described, but several different ones may coexist in the same patient: reticular, plaque-like, papular, atrophic, erosive and bullous, the latter being extremely rare. Often the condition is asymptomatic, but some complain of extreme soreness, especially with eating.

Where there is soreness, the use of *Myrrh* mouthwashes is helpful. Perhaps the key remedy in treatment is *Arsenicum album* 6–12 twice daily, especially in fastidious or fussy individuals. Failing that, *Natrum phosphoricum* 6–30 twice daily may be given. In erosive or atrophic forms, *Sulphur* 6–12 twice daily should be strongly considered. Otherwise, selection of a remedy based strongly upon the mental and general aspects of the patient may be helpful.

See also *Lichenoid reactions*.

Lichenoid reactions

These may be clinically indistinguishable from *lichen plants*, but asymmetry and palatal involvement are more typical of lichenoid reaction. The cause is generally a systemic drug, but *amalgam* reaction may also be responsible. The best treatment is for the physician to stop the particular drug or switch to another therapy, or for the dental surgeon to remove any offending amalgam restorations and replace them with other materials, whichever is appropriate. Drug-related cases will usually resolve within 3 months and those related to amalgam in a few weeks. Any oral soreness is best treated with *Myrrh* mouthwashes.

See also *AIDS; Anti-inflammatory drugs; Diabetes mellitus; Rheumatoid arthritis*.

Linear IgA disease

This uncommon disease, which produces non-specific oral *ulceration,* is probably a variant of *dermatitis herpetiformis*, and may be treated similarly. Skin lesions occur mainly on the buttocks, elbows and scalp.

Lingua villosa – *see* Tongue, black hairy

Lingual nerve injury – *see* Nerve injury

Lip, cracked – *see* Angular cheilitis; Lip, median fissure of lower

Lip, median fissure of lower

This is often infected with staphylococci, and is often persistent without treatment. A *Propolis* cream or ointment (Ø 20 drops in 50g of base) should be applied 3–6 times daily. *Natrum muriaticum* 6–12 three times daily is probably the key internal remedy, especially in hot individuals. *Sepia* 6–12 twice daily is better indicated in chilly types. Either *Pulsatilla* or *Chamomilla* may be used similarly, and should be prescribed according to susceptible typological indications.

Lueticum (Syphilinum)

A nosode of syphilis. A remedy occasionally used in the treatment of *exostoses*, and usually given infrequently. It may be helpful in the treatment of *Paget's disease*. An indented *tongue* is a partial indication for this remedy.

Lupus erythematosus

Two types of this disorder are described; discoid (DLE) and systemic (SLE). The oral signs of the two types are indistinguishable. The buccal and labial mucosae are usually involved bilaterally. There may be atrophic areas with peripheral erythema and white striae. The lesions must be distinguished from *lichen planus*. A butterfly erythematous rash of the face occurs in SLE. *Xerostomia* as part of *Sjögren's syndrome* occurs in about 30% of patients with SLE. *Myrrh* mouthwashes are helpful in controlling oral soreness. Homoeopathic treatment of the underlying disorder is complex.

Lycopodium (Lycopodium clavatum)*

Homoeopathic club moss spores. Useful in some cases of migraine, orofacial *neuralgia, tension headaches* and *xerostomia*, according to the typology. An important constitutional remedy. **Susceptible typology:** intelligent, difficult character, ill-tempered, thin, withered, yellowish and lined face, eyes lively, prematurely grey, looks older than he/she should, underlying profound anxiety and lack of confidence, one foot hot and the other cold, complaints dominantly right-sided or move from right to left, dyspeptic, desire for sweet things, < between 4pm and 8pm, < heat, > fresh air, prone to kidney stones.

Lyme disease

This disease, named after the town of Old Lyme in Connecticut (USA), is caused by the spiochaete Borrelia burgdorferi. It is transmitted by ticks (largely found in forests and woods), and is now widely distributed throughout Europe and the USA. It is also found in Australia. The first stage of the disease involves the development of a characteristic ring-like expansive rash around the site of the tick bite, termed erythema chronicum migrans, and the generation of an influenza-like illness. The second stage, which may occur from weeks to months after the first stage, may be associated with something resembling *Bell's palsy*, other neurological signs, cardiac abnormalities and skin rashes. The third stage of the disease, occurring months to years later, is characterised by a chronic

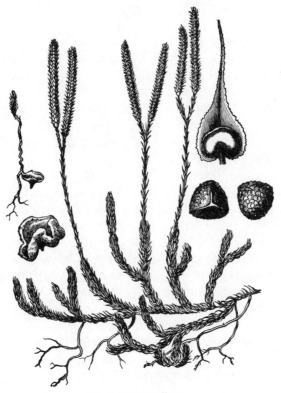

Fig. 26. Lycopodium

arthritis. Both orthodox and homoeopathic therapies are available. *Causticum* may be helpful in *facial nerve palsy* of the second stage.

Lymphangioma

This is a benign lesion, usually found upon the tongue of a child. It is probably developmental in origin. *Thuja* 6 twice daily may be tried.

Lymphogranuloma venereum

This venereal chlamydial disease is fairly widespread, and is characterised by an evanescent primary genital lesion (often unnoticed), inguinal buboes with sinus formation, and proctitis and rectal stricture in women and homosexual males. The primary lesion, a small herpetiform *ulcer*, may occasionally be seen on the tongue, with bubonic involvement of the submandibular lymph nodes.

M

Magnesia phosphorica

Homoeopathic magnesium phosphate. A remedy for trigeminal *neuralgia,* where the pain comes in severe and abrupt spasms, sometimes making the patient squeal or scream; predominantly right-sided, > heat and < cold. A remedy for the relief of muscular spasm > heat in cases of *craniomandibular dysfunction*. 'Mag. phos.', as it is termed, is best indicated in persons of *Phosphorus* **typology**. It may also be used to facilitate cranial *osteopathy*.

Magnesium

It has been suggested that magnesium supplementation may increase alveolar bone density. This is of some relevance in the treatment of chronic *periodontitis*, and the maintenance of the alveolar ridge in *prosthetics*. Magnesium amino acid chelate, a readily absorbable form of magnesium, provides 10–18mg of this element in 100mg of chelate. Daily supplementation is up to 1.67g of chelate.

See also *Calcium; Evening primrose oil*.

Mapped tongue – see Geographic tongue

Marble bone disease – see Osteopetrosis

Marfan's syndrome

This hereditary disease is characterised by bilateral subluxation of both lenses of the eye, congenital heart disease, weak musculature and long thin hands and feet. It is associated with recurrent *dislocation* of the TMJ.

Measles (Rubeola)

The first sign of measles may be witnessed by the dental surgeon. About 2 days before the main rash occurs, Koplik's spots appear in the mouth of a vaguely unwell patient. These last 1–4 days. They resemble table salt crystals (on a red base), are found on the buccal mucosa, and are absolutely diagnostic of measles, and no other disease. At this stage, *Pulsatilla* is the remedy which should be strongly considered.

Median rhomboid glossitis

This characteristically presents in the midline towards the back of the tongue. It is usually a reddened area, but is sometimes proliferative, and even superficial *ulceration* can occur. Once thought to be a developmental abnormality, it is now known that many cases are examples of oral *candidosis*. Initially it may be treated with the local and internal methods suggested in the entry relating to the latter. However, should these fail, the following remedies may be considered according to susceptible typology, and given in 6–12c twice daily: *Argentum nitricum, Arsenicum album, Causticum, Chamomilla, Kali bichromicum, Phosphorus* or *Rhus toxicodendron.*

See also *AIDS.*

Melanoma, malignant – see Pigmentation, oral & circumoral; Tumours & cysts

Melkersson-Rosenthal syndrome

The term given to the triad of facial swelling, deeply fissured *tongue* and recurrent *facial nerve palsy*. It has been regarded as a variant of *orofacial granulomatosis*. Treatment should be along the lines appropriate to the latter, in combination with those suggested for *Bell's palsy*.

Meniscus, disorders of TMJ – see TMJ, disorders of

Mercurius corrosivus

Homoeopathic corrosive sublimate. A remedy for *cancrum oris,* chronic *gingivitis* and *periodontitis, pemphigus* and *pemphigoid.*

Mercurius solubilis (Mercurius solubilis Hahnemannii) *

Homoeopathic dimercurous ammonium nitrate, a compound devised by Hahnemann. The properties are virtually identical to those of Mercurius vivus, metallic mercury. A remedy for dental *abscess, pericoronitis*, infant *teething, pulpitis*, chronic *gingivitis, periodontitis, mumps* (and other forms of acute viral parotitis), *ranula*, perversion of *taste, halitosis, ANUG*, and *sialorrhoea*. Its local indications are the combination of severe halitosis and excessive salivation, especially if the *tongue* bears the imprint of the teeth. **Susceptible typology:** flabby, sweaty, smelly, pungent bodily odour, splutters when speaking, < cold, < extreme cold or heat. The psychological type is variable. It may be the person who is slow in comprehension; one who is morose, timid and anxious; or the delinquent, recidivist, roguish wheeler and dealer, sexual pervert or obsessive voyeur.

See also *Appendix 2.*

***Mercury toxicity** – see* **Appendix 2**

***Methotrexate therapy** – see* **Folate**

Mezereum (Daphne mezereum)

Homoeopathic daphne mezereum. A remedy for *impetigo*, where a thick yellow pus exudes from under a thick crust. Also indicated in some cases of *pulpitis* and *ranula*.

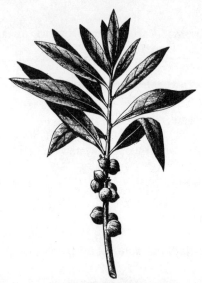

Fig. 27. Mezereum

***Migraine** – see* **Neuralgia, (periodic) migrainous**

***Migrainous neuralgia, periodic** – see* **Neuralgia, (periodic) migrainous**

Millefolium

Homoeopathic yarrow. It is indicated in dental *haemorrhage* where the blood is bright red, especially if there is an absence of pain and anxiety.

***Morphology, dental** – see* **Calcarea carbonica; Calcarea fluorica; Calcarea phosphorica**

Mottling – *see* **Fluoridation; Fluorosis**

Mouth, burning – *see* **Burning mouth syndrome**

Mouth-breathing

This is frequently due to nasal catarrh with enlarged adenoids in children. In some cases, food allergy is a contributory factor, the most common allergen in this respect being cow's milk; the elimination of this and its products producing considerable improvement within several months. Otherwise, homoeopathic remedies may be selected on the basis of the susceptible typology, the most important of which are: *Agraphis nutans, Calcarea phosphorica, Calcarea carbonica, Pulsatilla* and *Sulphur*. The selected remedy may be given initially in 6–12c twice daily. Infrequent doses of *Bacillinum* or other major nosodes may be occasionally required.

Mouthwashes

The most important are those of *Calendula, Myrrh* and *Propolis. Hydrastis* mouthwash is worthy of consideration, as is that of kitchen (garden) sage, Salvia officinalis (see *Aphthous ulcers*).

See also *Aloe vera; Berberis vulgaris; Folate; Zinc*.

Mucocele

This lesion of the minor salivary glands may be caused by trauma or duct obstruction, and is most commonly seen on the inner aspect of the lower lip. Mucoceles usually have the pattern of alternating rupture and reappearance. Some respond well to *Silicea* 6–12 twice daily.

Mucormycosis – *see* **Fungal diseases**

Multiple sclerosis

Some cases manifest *trigeminal neuralgia*. The occurrence of the latter in a person under 40 years of age is suggestive of multiple sclerosis or *AIDS*.

Mumps

One type of viral swelling of the *salivary glands*. It may affect both the parotid and the submandibular glands. Sometimes the latter alone are involved. The key remedies are *Jaborandi* and *Pulsatilla*.

See also *Salivary glands, viral infections of*.

Myristica

Homoeopathic preparation of the poisonous gum obtained by incising the bark of Myristica sebifera (known as Ucuuba in Brazil, and related to the nutmeg tree). A remedy for acute dental *abscess* with obvious swelling of the soft tissues. It may be also useful in the treatment of *cellulitis*.

Myrrh

Botanic. An oleo-gum-resin obtained from the stems of various species of Commiphora. The mother tincture is usually diluted to produce a *mouthwash*: Ø 5ml plus water 45ml. This is useful for reducing soreness and inflammation in the mouth, and may be used in a variety of conditions, such as *aphthous ulcers*, atrophic or erosive *lichen planus*, other *ulcerative* conditions, *gingivitis* or *periodontitis*.

N

Naevus, white sponge – see **Sponge naevus, white**

Natrum carbonicum

Homoeopathic sodium carbonate. A remedy for *tension headache* brought on by hot weather, especially in those who are weak, hypersensitive to sudden noises, prone to recurrent sprains and feel chilly in the winter.

*Natrum muriaticum**

Homoeopathic rock salt (crude sodium chloride). Useful in some cases of *halitosis, burning mouth syndrome, herpes labialis, aphthous ulcers*, puberty or pregnancy *gingivitis, epulis, ranula, geographic tongue*, median fissure of the *lip*, atypical *facial pain*, migraine or migrainous *neuralgia, tension headache*, perversion of *taste* (salty), black hairy *tongue, Sjörgren's syndrome* and *xerostomia*. A major constitutional remedy. **Susceptible typology:** depressive, weak, pale, thin, dislikes and rejects consolation, difficult concentration, greasy face, dryness of mucous membranes, strong desire for salt, thirsty, chilly but dislikes hot weather or hot rooms, prone to headaches, < at the seaside.

Natrum phosphoricum

Homoeopathic sodium phosphate. A remedy for *lichen planus,* especially in cases that exhibit a yellow creamy coating towards the back of the *tongue*.

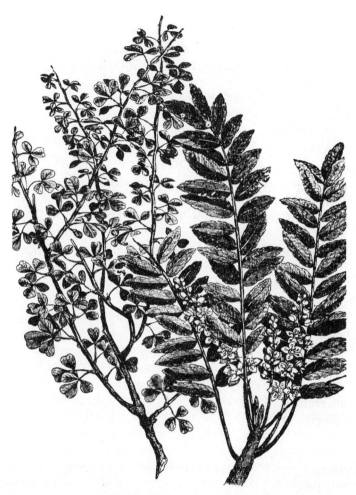

Fig. 28. Myrrh & Frankincense

Necrotising sialometaplasia

This unusual condition classically occurs on the palate, and may follow trauma, such as that from local *anaesthesia*. Preceding its onset there may be an episode of greater palatine nerve anaesthesia or paraesthesia. It may resemble squamous cell *carcinoma* both clinically and histologically. However, unlike the more serious lesion, it will resolve within 14 days, recurrence being rare. Only *Myrrh* or *Calendula* mouthwashes are required for treatment.

Needle, broken hypodermic – see Foreign body

Nerve injury

For injury to sensory nerves (e.g. the lingual nerve), *Hypericum* 6–30 three times daily promotes regeneration and restoration of sensation. For injury to motor nerves (e.g. the facial nerve), *Causticum* 6–30 three times daily is preferable, although Hypericum may be tried. Neither remedy is capable of any effect if there is considerable misalignment of the severed section of nerve.

Neuralgia, glossopharyngeal

This is a very similar disorder to trigeminal neuralgia. However, the pain is often brought on by swallowing, and may be felt in the ear, throat or larynx. *Acupuncture* combined with the administration of *Scutellaria* Ø may be helpful. The selection of homoeopathic remedies is best based upon the constitutional aspects of the case, rather than those of the presenting complaint. *Thuja* is worthy of consideration in some cases.

See also *Neuralgia, trigeminal.*

Neuralgia, (periodic) migrainous (Cluster headache/Facial migraine)

Under this heading, it is practical to consider three related entities: migraine, periodic migrainous neuralgia and paroxysmal hemicrania. Although it is now claimed that migraine should be considered as a separate entity from migrainous neuralgia, partially upon the basis that the appropriate orthodox therapies are different, it is a fact that, as many migraine sufferers (particularly women) approach middle-age, the pain shifts downwards to the face. I do not mean to imply, however, that migrainous neuralgia is purely a condition of females over 30, for it may also be experienced by those of younger years and either sex, even without a history of migraine as such; although many will report that they have suffered from recurrent headaches in the past. There is also, in many instances, some diagnostic confusion between migrainous neuralgia and *craniomandibular dysfunction* (TMJ dysfunction syndrome), with the patient presenting with symptoms of both. This turns out, however, to be more of a problem for the orthodox practitioner than he or she who is more homoeopathically inclined; for, homoeopathy and allied natural therapies are more readily applied to patients who cannot be categorised conventionally.

Migraine is classically defined as a unilateral headache accompanied by visual disturbance and nausea. It often lasts for many hours. Some-times the visual disturbance (often fortification spectra) is manifest alone. Attacks may be precipitated by such foods as cheese, red wine and chocolate, and many are related to stress. The dental surgeon may become intimately involved in such cases, since the provision of upper or lower acrylic splints (bite-plates) has been found helpful in many cases. These should only be worn at night. However, manipulation of the thoracic and cervical spine, as mentioned in the section on cranio-mandibular dysfunction, is also most useful in many instances. *Acupuncture* is also an excellent technique not to be forgotten. Where the migraines occur on almost a daily basis, 'occult' *food allergy* is to be suspected. This diagnosis is unlikely in the infrequent case. The com-monest allergens in this respect are cow's milk and wheat, the supervised exclusion of which is relatively simple. Related to the matter of food allergy, is sugar sensitivity. These patients suffer from what is termed 'clinical hypoglycaemia', and improve considerably when sweets, sugar, chocolates, cakes and biscuits are removed from the diet and they can be persuaded to take extra snacks between main meals. Where stress is involved, the *Bach flower remedies* are useful. Homoeopathic constitu-tional remedies may also be usefully given, based upon the generals and mentals of the case. In women, migraine may be associated with hormonal disturbances, and remedies such as *Natrum muriaticum, Pulsatilla* and *Sepia* stand high on the list of remedies to be considered. *Evening primrose oil* may also improve such cases. The botanic medicine *Feverfew*, taken in the form of capsules or tablets, has acquired a strong reputation for the prevention and treatment of migraine in general. Some patients, however, develop oral *ulceration* as a result, and the medicine must be discontinued.

Periodic migrainous neuralgia is characterised by a severe unilateral pain around the eye, in the temple or in the cheek, lasting from 30 to 120 minutes. During the attack, the affected side becomes flushed, and there may be conjunctival injection, lacrimation and rhinorrhoea. A particular characteristic, in some cases, is the precipitation of an attack by even tiny amounts of alcohol of any sort. This is one of the few non-dental pains which will cause patients to awake prematurely. In general, it is episodic, and there may be days or weeks between attacks. However, there are some cases in which the pain, which is often described as 'burn-ing', occurs with greater frequency, sometimes on an almost daily basis. Paroxysmal facial hemicrania is essentially similar to migrainous neuralgia, but lacks the facial flushing, lacrimation, rhinorrhoea and the provocation of waking. Moreover, the attacks are often shorter, lasting up to 20 minutes. Some of these cases are far from paroxysmal, and the pain, which is often throbbing and jabbing, may be virtually continuous. It is then a matter of argument whether they should be classified as craniomandibular dysfunction or facial hemicrania. The pain of this variant of facial hemicrania is more severe that that of atypical *facial pain*.

Apart from the total exclusion of alcohol in some cases, the treatment of both migrainous neuralgia and paroxysmal facial hemicrania has many features in common with that for craniomandibular dysfunction or migraine. Manipulation of the thoracic and cervical spine is often helpful, particularly in the C7/T1 area, along with acupuncture, especially to Stomach 6. With frequent or almost continuous attacks, food allergy or sugar sensitivity may be suspected. The application of Bach flower or homoeopathic constitutional remedies and evening primrose oil is similar. Additionally, remedies may be prescribed pathologically, their selection being largely determined by the individualised symptoms of the presenting complaint, including its laterality. This is a useful method for the practitioner who is not expert in constitutional prescribing, which is the alternative approach. The remedies to be looked at particularly in this respect are: *Apis mellifica*, *Aranea diadema*, *Carbolicum acidum*, *Iris versicolor*, *Kali bichromicum*, *Kalmia latifolia*, *Paris quadrifolia*, *Sanguinaria canadensis* and *Spigelia* . The selected remedy may be prescribed preventatively in 6–30c twice daily, or may be used to abort an attack, giving it in 30–200c every 15–30 minutes.

Neuralgia, post-herpetic

Persistent neuralgia following an attack of herpes zoster (shingles) is usually preventable and treatable by means of remedies. The key remedy is *Kali phosphoricum* 6–30 two or three times daily. Should this fail (which is unlikely), consider *Hypericum* 30 three times daily. Resistant cases may require infrequent doses of Varicella nosode 30–200. Oral *vitamin E* supplementation and injections of *vitamin B12* are also sometimes used in therapy.

See also *Herpes zoster*.

Neuralgia, trigeminal (Prosopalgia/Tic douloureux)

This unilateral pain may involve any division of the trigeminal nerve. Its fundamental characteristic is its utmost severity, the pain often being described as 'lancinating', 'shooting' or 'knife-like'. It usually occurs in attacks and bouts. Bouts of pain, consisting of numerous attacks, may last for weeks or months, between which the patient is asymptomatic. These then recur. An attack during a bout of trigeminal neuralgia may be brought on by cold draughts, eating, talking or touching certain trigger points. This disorder seldom occurs in patients younger than 40 years of age, and its occurrence in those younger is suggestive of an underlying disorder, such as *multiple sclerosis* or *AIDS*. Neoplasms of the nasopharynx or maxillary antrum, acoustic neuromata and aneurysms may be rarely associated with trigeminal neuralgia. The term 'pre-trigeminal neuralgia' refers to symptoms which occur before the onset of the overt disorder. There may be a recurrent mild or moderate pain, which is confused with such entities as *pulpitis* and *cervical sensitivity*; or there may be a 'crawling' sensation on the skin of the face.

Fortunately, results with acupuncture can be most satisfying, including the use of multiple facial needles on the *opposite* side to that of the pain. In conjunction, I feel that *Scutellaria* Ø, 5–10 drops in water three times daily, is helpful. Homoeopathic remedies are best prescribed on a constitutional basis, with the main emphasis being placed upon the generals and mentals, rather than any great emphasis being alloted to the presenting symptoms. Laterality, however, may be useful in the repertorisation of the case, and in this regard it is interesting to note that more cases are right-sided rather than left. Alternatively, remedies may be prescribed largely on the basis of the individualised symptoms, and this approach may be useful in cases where the constitutional simillimum is difficult to define. In this respect, the following remedies warrant special consideration: *Aranea diadema, Carbolicum acidum, Cinnabaris, Hypericum, Kalmia latifolia, Magnesia phosphorica, Paris quadrifolia, Prunus spinosa, Rhododendron chrysanthum, Spigelia* and *Verbascum*. The selected remedy may be prescribed in 6–30c two or three times daily. The use of *Thuja* in obstinate cases is sometimes worthy of consideration.

Niacin – see **Pellagra**

Nicotinamide – see **Pellagra**

Nitricum acidum (Acidum nitricum)
Homoeopathic nitric acid. A remedy for diarrhoea following *antibiotics, ANUG, ecthyma contagiosum, ranula, halitosis* and *aphthous ulcers*. Pricking pains are a characteristic indication for its use in the latter. **Susceptible**

typology: essentially similar to that of *Sepia*, but with a desire for fatty food. The presence of a fissured tongue is a leader to this remedy.

Noma – *see* Cancrum oris

Nosebleed – *see* Epistaxis, acute

Nux vomica*

Homoeopathic poison nut, which contains strychnine. Useful in some cases of migraine, migrainous *neuralgia, xerostomia, halitosis, tension headache*, and perversion of *taste*, depending on typological indications. A major constitutional remedy, which, as with others, may be useful in the treatment of chronic *periodontitis*, provided that the generals and mentals match the case. **Susceptible typology:** the overworked business man or professional, the person with a sedentary occupation, depressive, irritable, chilly, dyspeptic, prone to peptic ulcer and headaches, prone to constipation and haemorrhoids (which are > cold baths), prone to overindulgence in alcohol and rich foods, sleepy after meals, insomnia at night, hungover and sneezing in the morning, tongue coated white posteriorly, sometimes with varicose sublingual veins.

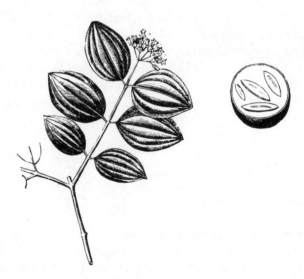

Fig. 29. Nux vomica

O

***Odontalgia, atypical (Atypical odontogenic pain) – see* Facial pain, atypical**

***Odontophobia – see* Anxiety, acute dental**

Opium
Homoeopathic opium. A remedy for speeding the arousal of those who have been the subject of general *anaesthesia*. Some recommend *Phosphorus* as an alternative.

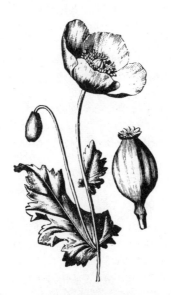

Fig. 30. Opium poppy

***Oral contraceptives – See* Contraceptives, oral**

Oral surgery, pain control after (including that related to periodontal surgery, extraction & apicectomy)
Arnica 30–200 is routinely used to control bleeding, bruising and pain of traumatised soft tissues. For pain at the site of an incision, *Staphysagria* 30–200 is better indicated, and can be more effective than morphine in many instances. This remedy also promotes epithelial repair. For bone or periosteal pains, *Ruta* 30–200. For shooting nerve pains, consider

Hypericum 30–200. Any of these remedies may be repeated with great frequency initially, in order to control pain, e.g. every 15–30 minutes. The frequency should be reduced as the pain improves and the tissues enter the healing phase.

In many instances, the routine prescription of Arnica and Hypericum together, both before and after the procedure, in conjunction with post-operative *Calendula* formentations or *mouthwashes*, will suffice to keep discomfort and pain to a tolerable minimum.

See also *Anaesthesia, local; Fracture, jaw.*

Oral surgery, prevention of complications in

In this respect, consult the appropriate sections: *Arnica; Anaesthesia, general; Anaesthesia, local; Antimonium tartaricum; Calendula; Fracture, jaw; Haemorrhage, acute dental; Hypericum; Opium; Pyrogen; Subacute bacterial endocarditis, prevention of.*

Also remember that healing requires adequate amounts of nutritional materials, and that those slow to heal may lack one or more essential substances.

See *Vitamin A; Vitamin C; Vitamin E; Zinc.*

Orf – see Ecthyma contagiosum

Orofacial granulomatosis (OFG)

The clinical oral manifestations of OFG are very similar to those of *Crohn's disease*: *angular cheilitis*, swelling of the lip, buccal mucosal thickening (cobblestone appearance), full width *gingivitis*, oral ulceration and mucosal tags, mainly of the retromolar area. Unlike Crohn's disease, the clinical involvement is normally restricted to the orofacial region. It is believed that most cases are due to orofacial *allergy*, the most likely allergens being cinnamon, benzoic acid (a common preservative) and chocolate. Most cases resolve within 18 months of removal of the appropriate allergen or allergens. Local treatment with *Myrrh* or *Propolis* may be helpful. Infrequent doses of *Bacillinum* are sometimes indicated.

See also *Melkersson-Rosenthal syndrome.*

Orofacial pain – see Facial pain

Orthodontics

Mechanical trauma to the oral mucosa from appliances is best treated with *Calendula* cream, ointment or *mouthwashes*. Oral *candidosis* may occasionally occur, the treatment of which is discussed under the appropriate section. The prescription of either *Calcarea fluorica* or *Calcarea phosphorica* 6–12 twice daily, according to the dominant dental morphology, is useful for facilitating movement (the greater the asymmetry, the better indicated is Calcarea fluorica). Given concurrently or independently, *Ruta* 6–12 twice daily assists in the repair of the periodontal ligament, and reduces the discomfort of orthodontic pressure.

See also *Sialorrhoea*.

Oscillococcinum

An homoeopathic nosode prepared from duck tissue infected with an oscillating organism. Used primarily in the prevention and treatment of *colds and influenza*.

Osteitis deformans – *see* Paget's disease

Osteogenesis imperfecta

A congenital abnormality of bone formation, where a *fracture* may occur with trivial force, associated with a peculiar blue colour of the sclerotic coat of the eye. Recurrent *dislocation* of the jaw may occur. Dentino-genesis imperfecta, where the dentine is imperfectly formed, may occur. Some cases only manifest the defect of the dentine together with the blue sclera. *Calcarea phosphorica* and *Symphytum* are indicated.

Osteoma

Some respond to *Calcarea fluorica* 6–12 twice daily. Infrequent doses of *Lueticum* may also be required. *Oral surgery* may be indicated, with the usual precautionary homoeopathic methods.

See also *Fluorosis; Torus mandibularis & palatinus*.

Osteomyelitis

Remedies such as *Phosphorus, Hekla lava* or *Amphisbaena* (6–30c 4-hourly) should be considered according to indications, the selected remedy being given in conjunction with *Pyrogen* 30 three times daily. *Silicea* 6–12 three times daily promotes the expulsion of sequestra.

Osteopathy

A school of manipulative therapies allied to chiropractic, of which cranial osteopathy is a particular sub-speciality. Useful in the treatment of migraine and migrainous *neuralgia, carpal tunnel syndrome, tension headache* and *craniomandibular dysfunction.*

See also *Magnesia phosphorica.*

Osteopetrosis (Albers-Schönberg disease/ Marble bone disease)
A rare disease of bone, usually of congenital origin. It is characterised by extreme bone density, susceptibility of bone to infection (as a result of diminished blood supply) and secondary anaemia. Fractures occur with minimal trauma due to abnormalities of collagen and mineral salt distribution. *Osteomyelitis* may occur in the jaws. *Calcarea fluorica* and *Symphytum* may be useful in fundamental therapy.

Osteoporosis – see Calcium

Osteosarcoma – see Fluorosis; Tumours & cysts

Osteosclerosis – see Fluorosis

P

Paget's disease (Osteitis deformans)
Compression of the branches of the trigeminal nerve in this condition results in oral and *facial pain.* Where the jaws are involved, the maxilla is more commonly affected. There is broadening of the alveolus and separation of the teeth. Extraction may be difficult because of *hyper-cementosis.* Homoeopathic treatment involves such remedies as *Aurum metallicum, Calcarea phosphorica, Hekla lava, Silicea* and *Lueticum.*

Pain – see Abscess, dental; Facial pain; Oral surgery, pain control after; Pain threshold, low; Pulpitis; Toothache

Pain threshold, low
This may be raised in those of appropriate typology by the judicious use of remedies, especially *Chamomilla* and *Coffea cruda,* 30–200.

See also *Anxiety, acute dental; Kali carbonicum.*

Palsy, Bell's – see Bell's palsy

Palsy (Paralysis), facial nerve – see Facial nerve palsy

Papilloma, squamous

This is a benign lesion of the mouth, with little likelihood of malignant change. Excision, together with the normal homoeopathic precautions of *oral surgery*, is the most expedient treatment. Otherwise, *Thuja* 6–12 twice daily may be tried.

See *Papillomavirus lesions, human.*

Papillomavirus lesions, human

There are many different types of human papillomavirus (HPV). Such viruses may be implicated in the development of squamous cell *papilloma, condyloma acuminatum, focal epithelial hyperplasia* (Heck's disease), *verruca vulgaris, leukoplakia* and squamous cell *carcinoma.* Papillomavirus lesions may be associated with *AIDS.*

Some papillomavirus lesions may be treated with *Thuja* 6–12 twice daily, with a satisfactory response. Certainly this is so with the benign types. Whether a similar approach is applicable to *leukoplakia* or squamous cell *carcinoma*, remains to be seen.

Paracoccidiomycosis (South American blastomycosis) – see Fungal diseases

Paris quadrifolia

Homoeopathic Herb Paris. A remedy for facial *neuralgia*. Burning, prickling, lancinating pains, especially of the left side and < touch. A sensation as if the eye were pulled backwards by a thread. **Susceptible typology:** nervous, excessively talkative, jumps incoherently from one subject to another (very similar to the *Lachesis* type).

Parodontal abscess – see Abscess, dental

Parotitis, chronic recurrent (of childhood) – see Sialectasis

Paroxysmal facial hemicrania – see Neuralgia, (periodic) migrainous

Pellagra

Niacin is the generic term for nicotinamide and other derivates of similar activity. Deficiency of niacin is often seen in alcoholics. Severe deficiency results in the triad of dermatitis, dementia and diarrhoea. This is termed pellagra. Intraorally, moderate or severe niacin deficiency is associated with *glossitis* and stomatitis. The tongue becomes painful, red and swollen, with hypertrophy of the papillae. Later, the papillae atrophy, with the development of a shiny and smooth surface on the tongue. The gingival component of the stomatitis is essentially similar to *ANUG*, perhaps with the involvement of the same bacteria. The oral mucosa may become the seat of oral *candidosis*. Treatment is with oral nicotinamide and other measures to control oral infection. Advanced pellagra is a potentially fatal disease.

Pemphigoid, mucous membrane
In this form of pemphigoid, mucosal lesions are common, but those of the skin are rare. They may be desquamative *gingivitis*, bullae and erosions within the mouth. The conjunctivae and genital mucosa may be affected. Referral to an ophthalmic specialist is always warranted. Local and homoeopathic treatment of this condition is along similar lines to those given for *pemphigus*.

See also *Ulcers*.

Pemphigus
This uncommon vesiculobullous disorder, which has four main subtypes, dominantly affects the middle-aged and elderly, and is potentially fatal without satisfactory treatment. Urgent referral to a specialist physician is thus warranted. Bullous lesions and erosions are found in the mouth and other mucosal sites, and skin lesions may occur. Locally, *Myrrh* or *Propolis* mouthwashes may be helpful. Homoeopathically, *Rhus toxicodendron* 6–12 three times daily may be considered for early cases, and *Arsenicum album* 6 three times daily for more established cases. Unresponsive cases may require *Mercurius corrosivus* 6 three times daily.

See also *Ulcers*.

Periapical abscess – *see* Abscess, dental

Periapical cyst – *see* Endodontics

Pericoronitis (Wisdom tooth infection)
Internal homoeopathic treatment essentially follows the same lines as for dental *abscess*. Long-term use of *Hepar sulph*, 6 three times daily may be required to control the condition until the wisdom tooth can be extracted. An alternative is *Cheiranthus* 30 three times daily, which is especially indicated if *trismus* is present. Local treatment includes

swabbing the pocket with *Propolis Ø*, and *Myrrh* or *Propolis* mouthwashes. See also *Glandular fever*.

Periodontal surgery – *see* **Oral surgery, pain control after; Oral surgery, prevention of complications in**

Periodontitis, acute traumatic – *see* **Traumatised tooth**

Periodontitis, chronic (formerly termed Pyorrhoea, in the presence of purulent exudate)

Under this heading will be considered the treatment of both common chronic gingivitis and common chronic periodontitis, in that they are essentially related conditions. Both, of course, may be subject to acute or subacute exacerbations. Any comments concerning therapy must be prefaced by stating that there is no real substitute for correct oral hygiene and regular *scaling and polishing*. Any nutritional or medicinal aids to therapy must be based firmly on these aspects. From the practical point of view, we may classify our measures into: dietetic, systemic supplementary, topical and homoeopathic.

The most satisfactory diet is one that is low in sugars, but high in fibre and fruit. Diets which are deficient in *calcium* or *magnesium* may contribute to alveolar bone loss.

A number of nutritional substances have been suggested as being of benefit in the treatment of gingivitis and periodontitis. Considered overall, their effect may be partially due to their direct action on the periodontal tissues, and partially due to plaque inhibition. These include: *vitamin A, vitamin C, bioflavonoids, vitamin E, selenium,* folic acid, *coenzyme Q10, zinc* and magnesium. Any or all of these may be considered in a particular case. However, since the effects of coenzyme Q10 can be quite remarkable, I suggest that it is given at the outset in most cases. Co-enzyme Q10 should not be given in pregnancy. A single dose of 30mg daily after food is adequate for most cases. Other supplements may be added subsequently according to lack of response or indications of deficiency (from the dietetic history, the general history, objective or subjective symptoms, and special tests). Zinc deficiency is extremely common, even without overt signs, especially in vegetarian patients. Whether *evening primrose oil* is of benefit to bone density in menopausal patients remains to be seen. Vitamin E is often well-indicated in smokers, should not be used in pregnancy without professional advice, and is contraindicated (as is evening primrose oil) in cases of breast cancer. Further details of indications and contraindications for various supplements are documented under the appropriate headings.

It has been shown that zinc *mouthwashes* may be beneficial. These, however, are so utterly revolting in taste that I would not inflict them upon my worst enemy. 0.1% folic acid mouthwashes are useful in those taking the contraceptive pill, hormone replacement therapy, phenytoin or methotrexate, and those who are pregnant (see *Gingivitis, pregnancy; Gingivitis, phenytoin; Folate*). *Myrrh* mouthwashes are of general use in most cases, particularly where there is an acute or subacute exacerbation of the condition.

Homoeopathic prescribing may be either pathological or constitutional, or a combination of these. Constitutional prescribing is based mainly on the general and mental aspects of the case, and there appear to be no particular dominant types associated with periodontal disease. Pathological prescribing, however, is mainly based on the details of the oral condition. Galgut gives us a useful list of remedies in this respect, together with their characteristic indications. These are quoted with some minor modifications. The leading indication for each remedy is given in **bold type**, and the confirmatory indications after:

(1) *Mercurius corrosivus*. **Subacute inflammation.** Redness, bleeding, pocketing, mobility.

(2) *Mercurius solubilis*. **Acute inflammation with marked salivation.** Peculiar *taste*, abscesses, purulent discharge from pockets, pain, *halitosis*.

(3) *Phosphorus*. **Chronic inflammation with much bleeding.** Dry mouth, no halitosis, smooth tongue.

(4) *Silicea*. **Long history of repeated abscesses.** Longstanding chronic destruction, many infra-bony defects, especially indicated in chilly people who lack self-confidence.

(5) *Kali carbonicum*. **Purulent pockets without abscesses.** Abundant saliva, *halitosis*, bad taste, tongue pale or coated, digestive upsets.

(6) *Cistus canadensis*. **Thin friable gums that bleed easily.** Mouth feels cold, especially indicated in chilly subjects.

(7) *Staphysagria*. **Bleeding with bone loss.** High *caries* rate, pain in non-carious teeth, black stained teeth.

(8) *Calcarea carbonica*. **Persistent oozing of blood.** Lips stained with blood in the morning, halitosis, sour taste, teeth ache, alternating bouts of dryness and salivation.

(9) *Calcarea fluorica*. **Teeth loosening in sockets.** Dry indurated tongue, pain and burning sensations, digestive problems.

(10) *Arsenicum album*. **Atrophic gingivitis.** Dry or *burning mouth,* wandering pains in teeth and jaws, concomitant drug therapy, especially indicated in worn out patients.

(11) *Natrum muraticum*. **Painful marginal gingivitis without bleeding.** Prone to *herpes simplex infection.*

(12) *Nitricum acidum*. **Atrophic gingivitis.** Especially around restorations or chrome prostheses (? *allergy*).

(13) *Thuja*. **Marked periodontitis with mouth ulcers.** Hyperplastic gingivitis, *epulis,* high decay rate, predisposition to root caries, intermittent burning sensations.

In general, the selected remedy may be given in 6–12c twice daily, and in conjunction with any appropriate local and supplementary therapies. It may be given for several weeks to months at a time, sometimes switching to treatments for the inhibition of dental *calculus.*

Another method of prescribing occasionally used is the administration of autonosodes. These are remedies prepared from infected material of the patient for whom they are solely intended. Gingival exudate, materia alba or calculus is collected and potentised. Generally, these autonosodes should be given infrequently (e.g. in a 6c, one dose morning and evening on a single named day each week, with no other remedy being given on that day). This therapy, which should be reserved for difficult or unresponsive cases, is usually given in conjunction with other indicated prescriptions, whether they be constitutional or pathological.

See also *AIDS.*

Perioral dermatitis

A condition similar to acne rosacea, but confined to the perioral region. The skin is red, with the presence of pustules or small papules. It may be associated with the use of topical steroid creams. Treatment follows the similar homoeopathic lines to those employed in acne rosacea, with *Sulphur* as a key remedy.

Perlèche – see Angular cheilitis

Pernicious anaemia – see Vitamin B12

Peutz-Jegher's syndrome

This inherited disorder is characterised by the presence of *pigmentation,* in the form of circumoral melanotic macules, and intestinal polyps.

Melanotic macules may also be distributed across the bridge of the nose. Recognition by the dental surgeon is important in that the intestinal polyps may occasionally undergo malignant transformation. Out of interest it should be mentioned that, apart from surgery, the nosode Medorrhinum figures prominently in the treatment of polyps at any site.

Pharmacy, the dental – *see* Appendix 1

Phenytoin therapy – *see* Folate; Gingivitis, phenytoin

Phosphorus*
Homoeopathic phosphorus. A remedy for dental *haemorrhage, gingivitis, periodontitis, burning mouth syndrome, median rhomboid glossitis, xerostomia* and *osteomyelitis*. It may be used to arouse patients after general *anaesthesia*. A major constitutional remedy. **Susceptible typology:** magnetic eyes, sociable, sentimental, talkative, interested in many things, may be a 'jack of all trades', enthusiastic, tends to hide depression which alternates with excitation, hidden fears, feels generally < before storms, depression or anxiety < at sunset, often tall and thin, < cold (but head symptoms, such as headaches, > cold), < lying on left side, burning pains, desires cold food and drinks, hungry, bleeds easily.
    See also *Dry socket*.

Phytolacca (Phytolacca decandra)
Homoeopathic poke-root. A remedy for *bruxism* or bruxomania in children whilst teething (compare *Cina*) and *halitosis*. In children, the principal indications are recurrent sore throats, the presence of enlarged and tender lymph glands, together with tooth-grinding in the eruptive phase. In adults, it is halitosis in subjects who have stiffness and pains over the whole body, < for cold and wet weather, > dry weather, but not > continued movement (compare *Rhus toxicodendron*).

Pigmentation, oral & circumoral
There are many causes for the presence of oral or circumoral pigmentation, including: racial skin pigmentation, *Addison's disease, amalgam tattoo,* oral *contraceptives,* antimalarials, tranquillisers, smoking, malignant *melanoma, fibrous dysplasia, AIDS,* and *Peutz-Jegher's syndrome*.

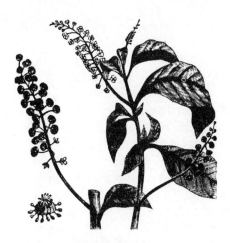

Fig. 31. Phytolacca

Plantago (Plantago major)

Homoeopathic greater plaintain. The mother tincture, locally applied, is an excellent therapy for *cervical sensitivity* and the sensitivity of a *chipped tooth*. It is also employed in the treatment of *dry socket*. The potentised remedy is useful in some cases of *pulpitis*. It may be used as a pulpal seditive when applied on cotton-wool to a carious or non-carious (lost filling) cavity.

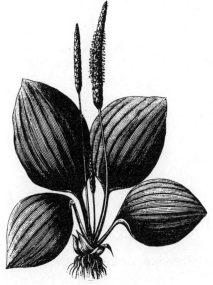

Fig. 32. Plantago

Pleomorphic salivary adenoma** – see **Salivary glands, neoplasms of

***Plummer-Vinson syndrome** – see* Iron

Podophyllum *(Podophyllum peltatum)*

Homoeopathic May Apple. A remedy for *bruxism*. It has been used to treat diarrhoea during *teething* and *sialorrhoea*. *Migraine* or *tension headache* relieved by diarrhoea is an indication. **Susceptible typology:** tendency to nausea (bilious temperament), prone to liver or biliary disease, diarrhoea from fresh fruit, *tongue* indented, tongue moist and thickly coated, bad *taste*, thirsty, prone to alternation between headache (or migraine) and diarrhoea.

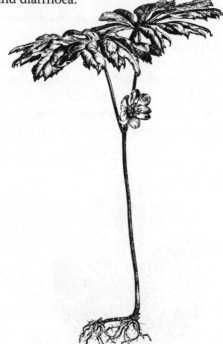

Fig. 33. Podophyllum

Pregnancy epulis** – see **Epulis

Pregnancy gingivitis** – see **Gingivitis, pregnancy

Progressive systemic sclerosis** – see **Scleroderma

Propolis

A substance produced by bees by the addition of saliva and wax to a resinous material gathered from the leaf buds and bark of poplars. It is anti-infective and anti-inflammatory. The mother tincture is exclusively used; undiluted, in aqueous dilution to varying degrees, or in the form of a cream or ointment. A satisfactory mouthwash may be prepared by adding 40–80 drops of Propolis Ø to 100ml of warm water. Propolis is used in the treatment of *ANUG, periocoronitis, herpes labialis,* pulpal *exposure, aphthous ulcers* and various other *ulcerative* conditions of the mouth, such as *pemphigoid* and herpetic *gingivostomatitis.*

Prosopalgia – *see* Neuralgia, trigeminal

Prosthetics, dental

Denture sore mouth is usually a manifestation of oral *candidosis.* The denture-bearing area is red, but is not necessarily sore. Allergy to acrylic or chrome appliances sometimes occurs, resulting in a form of this disorder with soreness. Allergy to denture material is also sometimes associated with *gingivitis, periodontitis* and *craniomandibular dysfunction.* Nutritional factors are probably important in the maintenance of the alveolar ridges.

See also *Angular cheilitis; Calcium; Denture granuloma; Evening primrose oil; Magnesium; Salivary glands, papillary or duct stricture of; Sialorrhoea.*

Prunus spinosa

Homoeopathic blackthorn flower buds. A remedy for *pulpitis,* facial *neuralgia* and opthalmic *herpes zoster.* It is indicated by pains in the eyes, as though they were about to explode, or neuralgic pains extending from the right side of the forehead to the occiput.

Ptelea

Homoeopathic water ash. A remedy for *sialorrhoea,* where food *tastes* bitter, especially in persons which chronic disorders of the stomach and liver (aching in liver region < lying on left side).

Ptyalism – *see* Sialorrhoea

Pulpitis, acute traumatic – *see* Traumatised tooth

Pulpitis

This is simply inflammation of the pulp, which may arise from *caries,* overheating or vibration from cavity preparation, mechanical exposure (from cavity preparation or fracture), 'concussion' of the pulp from a blow, or chronic irritation from an unlined restoration or *cervical sensitivity.*

(1) **Asymptomatic pulpitis.** This is associated with exposure of the pulp during cavity preparation, and may be accidental or inevitable, the latter being related to the removal of deep caries. A suitable dressing is of the calcium hydroxide type to which has been added a drop of *Propolis Ø. Belladonna* 6 three times daily should be given for three days in order to prevent progression of inflammation.

(2) **Mild symptomatic pulpitis following pulpal exposure and pulp-capping.** Fischer recommends *Hypericum* 30–200 initially at frequent intervals (every 30–60 minutes) to control the pain and inflammation following most exposures (including that related to fracture of a *traumatised tooth*). However, where the exposure is related to the excavation of deep caries and the pain < cold, he favours *Calcarea carbonica* 30–200 with similar repetition.

(3) **The vital tooth with minor pulpitic symptoms.** Here, there is usually excessive sensitivity to heat or cold, but the pain lasts for only a short time after stimulation (usually a few seconds, and seldom more than half a minute). Spontaneous pain, without any obvious provocation, is uncharacteristic, except with regard to the *traumatised* tooth. Tenderness to percussion is absent or mild. The key remedy is *Ferrum phosphoricum* 12–30 three times daily, which is especially indicated in thin or feeble patients. Should this fail, then give *Belladonna* 6–30 three times daily, which is most active in robust types. Either remedy may be complemented with *Pyrogen* 30 twice daily, if partial results are obtained. Pulpitis < before a period and > the flow is indicative of *Sepia* 6–12 twice daily.

(4) **Severe pulpitic symptoms.** Severe and prolonged toothache following thermal stimulation. Spontaneous pain, often severe, without overt stimulation. There may also be moderate tenderness on percussion, but this becomes more severe as pulp necrosis advances.

This type of tooth will generally require *endodontic* treatment or *extraction.* Remedies may be usefully given every 1–4 hours in order to control symptoms until either of the former can be instituted. Occasionally, however, the vitality of the pulp is fortuitously preserved, or the root canals become silently calcified. The indications for the various remedies are as follows:

(a) *Aconite* 30–200. Sudden onset of violent pain, often after cold air. Robust, young and active patients.

(b) *Belladonna* 30–200. Throbbing pain of sudden onset. Robust patients.

(c) *Ferrum phosphoricum* 12–30. Throbbing pain of sudden onset. Thin or feeble patients.

(d) *Arsenicum album* 6–30. Toothache ameliorated by warm water.

(e) *Mercurius solubilis* 6–30. Nightly aggravation of pain. Much salivation with halitosis.

(f) *Bryonia* 30–200. The pain increases progressively, reaches a peak, and disappears slowly. It is ameliorated by strong pressure on the tooth.

(g) *Plantago* 30–200. As with Mercurius solubilis, the pain is worse at night. The tooth is sensitive to the least contact, but paradoxically is > eating.

(h) *Mezereum* 30–200. This remedy has an elective action on the upper premolars and molars. Pain radiates to the temple or cheekbone, < eating, < least contact of tongue with tooth.

(i) *Apis mellifica* 30–200. Pain < heat and > cold. Especially indicated in those with the susceptible typology corresponding to *Natrum muriaticum* (depressive, greasy, thirsty, salt-loving types).

(j) *Coffea cruda* 30–200. Toothache > holding cold water in mouth. Especially indicated in patients intolerant of pain. Compare *Chamomilla* and *Clematis erecta*.

(k) *Prunus spinosa* 12–30. Toothache < hot foods, > clenching teeth. A sensation as though the tooth has been extracted.

The remedy *Hepar sulph.* should not be used in low potencies (e.g. 6c) for the treatment of pulpitis, since it may provoke abscess formation. However, used in 30–200c three times daily (or more often, according to the symptomatic response), it may abort pulpal necrosis, and preserve the vitality of the pulp, thus avoiding endodontic therapy. Its use should be reserved for cases unresponsive to a well-indicated remedy or where the selection of the simillimum is unclear.

In cases which have responded favourably to Belladonna, it is advisable to continue treatment with Calcarea carbonica 30 three times daily (or more frequently if necessary), after the severe throbbing pain has settled. Calcarea carbonica often follows well, and should be given until the tooth is rendered completely asymptomatic. A proportion of teeth treated in this manner undergo calcification of the root canals, thus removing the need for endodontic therapy.

It should be noted that pulpal sedation may be at least partially achieved by inserting Propolis Ø on cotton-wool into a carious or non-carious cavity. *Clove oil* is sometimes used similarly.

Pulsatilla (Pulsatilla nigricans) *

Homoeopathic European anemone. A remedy for *halitosis, gingivitis* of puberty, *mouth-breathing*, perversion of *taste*, migraine and migrainous *neuralgia, burning mouth syndrome; xerostomia,* median fissure of the lower *lip, mumps* and *measles*. A major constitutional remedy. **Susceptible typology:** timid, tearful, emotional, shy, placid, likes consolation, affectionate, often fair with blue eyes, skin of hands and feet mottled (venous stasis), thirstless, aversion to or < fats, < heat, indented *tongue*. Pulsatilla types often look younger than their years. However, it is also a remedy indicated in many elderly patients who are placid, timid, tearful, hot and thirstless. A yellow stripe down the centre of the tongue tends to support its applicability.

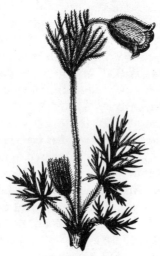

Fig. 34. Pulsatilla

***Puncture wound** – see* **Anaesthesia, local; Ledum**

***Pyogenic granuloma** – see* **Epulis**

***Pyorrhoea** – see* **Periodontitis, chronic**

Pyostomatitis vegetans

A non-specific pustular eruption which may be seen on the lips of those who suffer from either *Crohn's disease* or *ulcerative colitis*. Local treatment with *Calendula* or *Propolis* creams or ointments may be helpful.

Pyrethrum parthenium – see **Feverfew**

Pyrogen (Pyrogenium)

Homoeopathic nosode made from putrefying animal materials. Used in the control of sepsis and *septicaemia*. In *oral surgery*, Pyrogen 30 may be given twice daily to assist in the prevention of postoperative infection. This may be given along with other remedies normally used routinely, such as *Arnica* and *Hypericum*. It is occasionally used in the treatment of *dry socket* and *pulpitis*, in conjunction with other remedies.

See also *Abscess, dental; Cancrum oris; Osteomyelitis; Subacute bacterial endocarditis, prevention of.*

R

Radiography, ill-effects of

In order to combat the effects of ionising radiation, give a single dose of X-ray 30, preferably 30 minutes before taking X-rays.

Ramsay-Hunt syndrome

This condition arises from Varicella zoster infection of the geniculate ganglion. A unilateral *facial nerve palsy* develops, together with a homo-lateral vesicular cutaneous eruption of the external auditory meatus. The patient usually complains of pain in the region of the affected ear. Hyper-acusis may be present and oropharyngeal *ulceration*. Treatment should be commenced with *Causticum* 30 and *Rhus toxicodendron* 30 in 2-hourly alternation, decreasing the frequency of administration with improvement. Varicella nosode 30 may be given twice daily along with the previous treatment.

Supplementary therapies with *vitamin B12* and *vitamin E* should be given along the lines suggested for *herpes zoster*.

Ranula

This is a mucous retention cyst arising from one of the sublingual salivary glands, presenting as a large and often bluish swelling beneath one side of the tongue. The key remedies are *Ambra grisea* and *Calcarea carbonica*, followed by *Thuja* and *Mercurius solubilis*, depending on oral or susceptible typological indications. *Lachesis, Natrum muriaticum, Nitricum acidum, Mezereum* or *Staphysagria* may occasionally be required for obstinate cases. The selected remedy may be prescribed in 6–12c twice daily.

Reimplantation of tooth
Where a tooth has been completely dislocated from its socket, following retrograde *endodontic* technique, both should be irrigated with an aqueous dilution of *Propolis* Ø, 80 drops per 100ml normal saline/water. After fixation, in the case of both partial and complete dislocation, *Ruta* 6–30 three times daily should be given for many weeks, in conjunction with *Hepar sulph.* 6 three times daily. Also check the nutrition of the patient, especially with regard to *zinc* and *vitamin C* status, and supply supplementary doses if necessary. The remedy Silicea should not be given for any purpose before the tooth and the bone are satisfactorily reunited; otherwise, the tooth may be rejected.

See also *Traumatised tooth.*

Reiter's syndrome
This is characterised by the triad of arthritis, urethritis and *conjunctivitis.* The cause of the syndrome is uncertain, but some cases seem to be related to an episode of infective urethritis following sexual intercourse. Quite commonly, painful superficial *ulcers* appear on the palate, tongue and buccal mucosa. Local treatment may be given, as for *aphthous ulcers.* Internally, *Rhus toxicodendron* 30–200 two or three times daily is often indicated.

Rendu-Osler-Weber disease – *see* **Hereditary haemorrhagic telangiectasia**

Rescue Remedy – *see* **Bach flower remedies**

Rheum (Rheum officinale)
Homoeopathic rhubarb. A remedy for the child who is capricious and agitated whilst *teething*, where the whole child smells sour. Indicated in diarrhoea during teething.

Fig. 35. Rheum

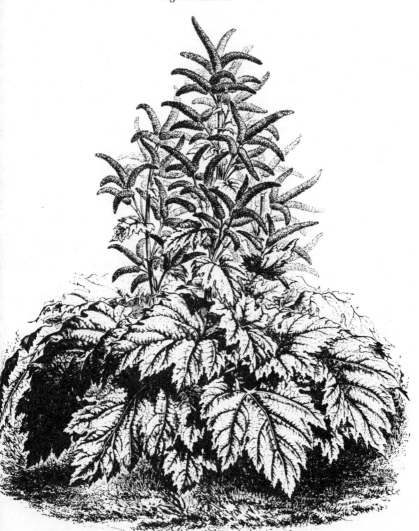

Rheumatoid arthritis

This may be associated with *iron* deficiency, leading to *aphthous ulcers* and oral *candidosis*. Anti-inflamatory drugs used in treatment may produce *lichenoid reactions*. Penicillamine therapy may cause distortion of *taste* and *vitamin B6* deficiency. Involvement of the *TMJ* may occasionally occur, leading to stiffness rather than pain. *Xerostomia* and *Sjögren's syndrome* may develop. Approximately half of the patients with

the combination of rheumatoid arthritis and Sjögren's syndrome are
allergic to the penicillin group of *antibiotics*.

See also *Zinc*.

Rhododendron chrysanthum

Homoeopathic Siberian rhododendron. A remedy for trigeminal *neuralgia*
brought on by stormy and thundery weather, and > after the storm. Also
< windy weather, and > dry heat.

Rhus toxicodendron

Homoeopathic poison ivy (from the river valleys of North America). The
mother tincture, whether diluted or undiluted, is unsuitable for intraoral use. A remedy for rheumatic or arthritic conditions which are
characterised by: < on initial movement, > for further movement, < prolonged movement, < in wet weather, > heat. Useful in some cases of
craniomandibular dysfunction and disorders of the *TMJ*. Also used in the
treatment of *ecthyma contagiosum, median rhomboid glossitis, pemphigoid,
pemphigus, herpes labialis, herpes zoster, Ramsay-Hunt syndrome, Reiter's
syndrome, xerostomia, Sjögren's syndrome,* jaw *fractures* and *chickenpox*.
Rhus toxicodendron is particularly effective in people who correspond to
the **susceptible typology** of *Phosphorus*. Great restlessness, especially
at night, also indicates its applicability, as does a coated tongue with a
red triangular area at the tip. An indented *tongue* is another indicative
feature.

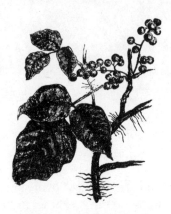

Fig. 36. Rhus toxicodendron

Riboflavine – *see* **Vitamin B2**

Root-filling – *see* **Endodontics**

Ruta (Ruta graveolens)

Homoeopathic rue. A remedy used in relation to *eye-strain*, *reimplantation* of dislocated teeth, jaw *fractures*, *orthodontics* and *sprain* of the wrist. A great remedy for the control of bone pain following any form of *oral surgery*. Used also in *endodontics* to control pain following apical penetration by a reamer, or apicectomy. It has been termed 'the *Arnica* of the periosteum'. A principal remedy for *dry socket*. Occasionally indicated in pain following local *anaesthesia*.

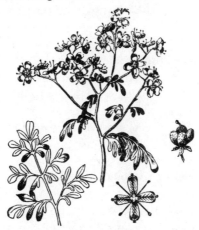

Fig. 37. Ruta

S

Salivary calculus (Sialolith/Salivary gland stone)

Calculi may develop in relation to any of the salivary glands, but those of the minor glands are clinically unimportant. Parotid calculi are nearly always found in the duct itself, whereas those of the submandibular gland are to be found either in the duct or within the substance of the gland. Since a large proportion of stones are radiolucent, they may be missed in routine radiography. Many are asymptomatic until duct obstruction occurs. Then, the usual presentation is intermittent swelling of the gland with some discomfort, particularly in relation to food. The initial treatment of choice is *Calcarea fluorica* 6–12 twice daily, a prescription which may need to be given for many months. Alterna-tively, *Lapis albus* 6 twice daily may be considered. Surgery may thus be avoided, even in intraglandular cases associated with recurrent episodes of acute bacterial sialadenitis (see below). *Silicea* 6–12 three times daily can induce the expulsion of stones obstructing the main parotid or sub-mandibular ducts, but is of doubtful use against intraglandular stones.

Salivary glands, bacterial infections of

This may occur as a result of calculi (see above), postoperative dehydra-tion, *sialectasis*, mucous plug, papillary or duct stricture (see after), cer-vicocranial radiotheraphy and *Sjögren's syndrome*. The swelling is acutely painful, and pus may discharge from the ductal orifice. *Calcarea fluorica* 12–30 three or four times daily is the initial treatment of choice. *Tuber-culosis* is a rare cause of chronic bacterial infection of the salivary glands.

Salivary glands, neoplasms of

Most parotid *tumours* are pleomorphic salivary adenomata (about 80%), some of which have responded well to *Lapis albus* 6–12 twice daily. Malignancy is more commonly associated with tumours of the sub-mandibular gland (about 60%), and virtually all those of the sublingual gland are sinister.

Salivary glands, papillary or duct stricture of

These sometimes are a consequence of trauma. In the case of papillary stricture, this may result from the teeth or a prosthesis. Symptoms are similar to those of *salivary calculus* with intermittent swelling of the gland in relation to food, and the remedy *Calcarea fluorica* may be employed similarly. Correction of any dental or *prosthetic* problems is necessary. Where Calcarea fluorica fails, long-term *Thiosinaminum* 6 twice daily should be considered. The buccinator window anomaly refers to a rare phenomenon, where spasm of this muscle occludes the parotid duct; again, Calcarea fluorica may be tried.

Salivary glands, viral infections of

A number of different viruses can affect the major salivary glands (*Cox-sackieviruses, influenza* viruses, echovirus, etc.), but the most important is *mumps*. Clinically, it may be impossible to distinguish between the different types of infection. However, from the homoeopathic point of view, treatment will often follow similar lines to that of mumps. Cytomegolovirus is a fairly harmless virus which may infect the salivary glands of the newborn or immunocompromised patients, such as those suffering from *AIDS*. This is known as cytomegalic or salivary gland inclusion disease.

Salivation, diminished – *see* Sjögren's syndrome; Xerostomia

Salivation, excessive – *see* Sialorrhoea

Sanguinaria canadensis

Homoeopathic blood root. A remedy for migraine and migrainous *neuralgia*. Pains are periodic, returning every seventh, third or second day. Predominantly right-sided. Cheek flushed. Burning or throbbing pain, < noise, < smell, < light, < movement, > resting in the dark, > passing wind (from above or below). Patients in whom it is indicated are generally thirsty, or menopausal with hot flushes. Sanguinaria canadensis extract is sometimes incorporated into botanic *toothpastes* for its beneficial action in cases of *gingivitis* or *periodontitis*.

Sarcoidosis

Clinical involvement of the oral mucosa in this disease, in which chronic granulomata develop in diverse sights, is extremely rare. The face or lips are more commonly involved, with the development of non-ulcerative plaques and nodules. Intermittent doses of *Bacillinum* have been used with good effect in some cases of sarcoidosis.

Scalds

These may be treated with *Hypericum* and *Calendula* ointment or cream, or with the oily contents of a *vitamin E* capsule.

Scaling & polishing

Bleeding and soreness may be controlled by using *Arnica* 30–200 three times daily, both before and after the procedure, together with either *Calendula* or *Myrrh* mouthwashes. Those who have *cervical sensitivity* should apply *Plantago* Ø before scaling.

See also *Calculus, dental; Subacute bacterial endocarditis, prevention of.*

Scar tissue, excessive

Keloid scars may be treated by giving a single dose of *Thuja* 30 once weekly on a particular day, and giving *Graphites* 6 twice daily on the remaining days. Additionally, Graphites 8x cream, to which *vitamin E*

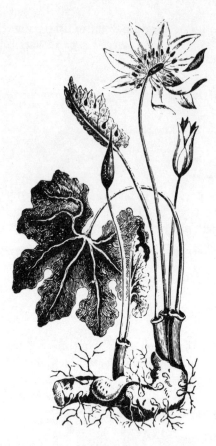

Fig. 38. Sanguinaria canadensis

has been added (600IU d-alpha tocopherol per 50g), should be applied two or three times daily.

In order to prevent or reduce excessive scar tissue associated with *oral surgery*, give *Thiosinaminum* 6 twice daily.

See also *Epidermolysis bullosa*.

Scleroderma (Progressive systemic sclerosis)

This is characterised by chronic sclerosis of the skin and vital organs. Involvement of the face leads to limitation of mouth opening. *Sjögren's syndrome* may develop. CREST syndrome is related to scleroderma, and consists of: *c*alcinosis, *R*aynaud's phenomenon, *o*esophageal stricture, *s*clerodactyly and *t*elangiectasia. Homoeopathic treatment for this condition is complex.

Scrofulous

An ancient adjectival term found in many old homoeopathic books of materia medica. It can be equated with a tendency to cervical lymphadenopathy.

Scutellaria (Scutellaria lateriflora)

Botanic. Skullcap. The mother tincture is sometimes used in the treatment of glossopharyngeal or trigeminal *neuralgia* and epilepsy.

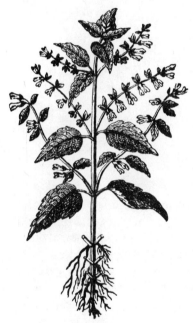

Fig. 39. Scutellaria

Selenium

This acts synergistically with *vitamin E*, and may be used in conjunction with it in the treatment of *gingivitis* or *periodontitis*. The usual daily dose is 200mcg. It is not recommended during pregnancy.

Sepia*

Homoeopathic cuttlefish ink. Indicated in median fissure of the lower *lip, herpes labialis, aphthous ulcers, pulpitis, xerostomia, burning mouth syndrome* and *gingivitis* of pregnancy or puberty. A major constitutional remedy, to be thought of in cases of atypical *facial pain*, periodic migraine and migrainous *neuralgia*, where the typology is appropriate. **Susceptible**

typology: often overworked housewives or business women, depressive with aggression to mainly their nearest and dearest, yet often the life and soul of the party, annoyed by consolation, uninterested in sex or abhorrence of sexual matters, weak memory, bored by many things, exhausted, very chilly, < before a storm, > vigorous exercise, desires acidic things, prone to constipation and haemorrhoids, bearing down feeling in pelvis, prone to varicose veins, indented *tongue, toothache* (pulpitis) < before periods and > the flow.

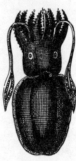

Fig. 40. Sepia

Septicaemia

This is, to some degree, preventable, and occasionally treatable with *Pyrogen* 30, given up to four times daily. It would be a better world if antibiotics were reserved for serious cases, or others where homoeopathic measures have failed. The use of antibiotics in cases of septicaemia is fully justified, and whilst the antibiotic may partially antidote the effect of the remedy, there is, nevertheless, good sense in giving Pyrogen concurrently.

Sequestrum

A small piece of non-vital bone remaining in the tissues after *oral surgery* may be expelled by giving *Silicea* 6–12 three times daily.

See also *Dry socket*; *Osteomyelitis*.

Shingles – *see* Herpes zoster

Sialectasis

Primary sialectasis is associated with chronic recurrent parotitis of childhood. Repeated attacks of suppurative bacterial sialadenitis occur in the parotid glands. The disease often resolves about puberty. Long-term treatment with *Calcarea fluorica* 6–12 twice daily may be helpful in

preventing acute exacerbations, and promoting resolution of the problem. Secondary sialectasis may be associated with chronic infection,
AIDS, irradiation or *Sjögren's syndrome*.

Sialolith – *see* Salivary calculus

Sialometaplasia, necrotising – *see* Necrotising sialometaplasia

Sialorrhoea (Ptyalism)

This may be associated with oral ulceration, such as primary herpetic
gingivostomatitis or *aphthous ulcers, diabetes mellitus* (diabetic autonomic
neuropathy), Parkinson's disease, cerebral palsy, mental retardation,
schizophrenia, epilepsy, *mercury* poisoning and various drug therapies.
In such cases, treatment or correction of the underlying cause is
helpful.

Some develop sialorrhoea when *orthodontic* or *prosthetic* appliances
are provided for the first time. In this respect, *Jaborandi 6–30* times daily
may be helpful. Other patients present with no obvious cause for the
sialorrhoea. Here, a variety of remedies may be useful. *Ptelea 6–30* twice
daily is indicated in those with chronic digestive or liver problems.
Mercurius solubilis 6–30 twice daily may be useful in those who have
severe halitosis and an indented tongue. For copious salivation after eating, especially in gluttonous and dyspeptic types, consider *Allium sativum*
6–30 three times daily. Also *Granatum* and *Podophyllum* are occasionally
indicated, according to typology. Podophyllum may be useful in the
drooling of old epileptics. Otherwise, constitutional prescribing, based
strongly upon the mentals and generals of the case, rather than details
of the presenting complaint, must be considered.

Sialosis

This is defined as a non-neoplastic, non-inflammatory enlargement of
the salivary glands. Bilateral parotid swelling is a common presentation,
but the other major salivary glands may also be affected. It is seen in
relation to *acromegaly,* alcoholism, malnutrition, *anorexia* and bulimia
nervosa, *diabetes mellitus* and a number of drug therapies. Treatment
of the underlying disorder usually results in some reduction of the
swelling.

Sicca syndrome – *see* Sjögren's syndrome

Silicea (Silica)*

Homoeopathic flint. A remedy for oroantral *fistula, mucocele,* black hairy *tongue,* delayed *eruption, xerostomia, osteomyelitis, actinomycosis, Paget's disease, salivary calculus* and *periodontitis.* Also used in *endodontics,* and for the expulsion of *foreign bodies* and a post-extraction *sequestrum.* To be used with caution in those with dental *implants* or where a tooth has been *reimplanted.* **Susceptible typology:** thin, weak, chilly, timid, nails have white spots (*zinc* deficiency), sweaty about head, smelly feet, prone to infection (wounds become infected readily), prone to cervical lymphadenopathy, < cold and draughts, < winter, > heat and dry weather, > summer, constipated with retraction of stool, prone to catarrhal disorders, prefers cold foods.

Sjögren's syndrome

The primary form of this disorder, formerly termed 'sicca syndrome', consists of diminished lacrimal and salivary secretion, leading to dry eyes and *xerostomia.* In the secondary form, the patient suffers from a connective tissue disorder in conjunction with dry eyes and/or xerostomia. Secondary Sjögren's syndrome is most frequently associated with *rheumatoid arthritis.* Less commonly it is found in relation to primary *biliary cirrhosis, scleroderma* or systemic *lupus erythematosus.* Enlargement of the salivary glands may occur in both types, but is not clinically apparent in the majority of cases. Secondary *sialectasis* and malignant lymphoma may occur in some cases of Sjögren's syndrome.

Natrum muriaticum 12–30 twice daily has been found helpful in a number of cases, resulting in an increase in lacrimal and salivary flow. *Rhus toxicodendron* 30–200 two or three times daily may be useful in cases associated with inflammatory arthritis. Other homoeopathic therapies may be required for the treatment of any concomitant connective tissue disorders.

Smelling salts

These contain ammonia and eucalyptus oil, the inhalation of which produces profound stimulation. They are an often forgotten, but important addition to the dental pharmacy. They are used in the treatment of simple *faint,* and dizziness following *local anaesthesia.*

Socket, infected tooth – see **Dry socket**

Spigelia

Homoeopathic Demerara pink-root. Used in some cases of *halitosis*. A remedy for trigeminal or migrainous *neuralgia*, particularly of the left side. Severe burning and prickling pains. Severe pains in the eyes as though they were too large, with flashing lights before them. Skin tender over affected side. Pain < movement, touch or shaking. Facial neuralgia < cold, > heat. Also a remedy for migraine or *tension headache* starting in the occiput and radiating to the left eye, which begins at dawn, increases in the day and diminishes by the evening. Paradoxically, the thermal modalities are opposite to those of the facial neuralgia. They are < heat and > cold. Spigelia is best indicated in weak and nervous patients, especially if they are prone to palpitations or are sensitive to changes in the weather. They tend to be prone to intestinal worm infestation.

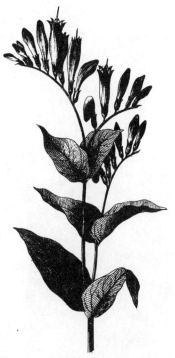

Fig. 41. Spigelia

Sponge naevus, white

This is an inherited abnormality, which is often first recognised in adolescence. Large areas of the oral floor and buccal sulcus are usually involved. Its appearance is similar to that of a repeatedly *bitten cheek*. The disorder is benign and warrants no special treatment. However, biopsy should be performed to differentiate it from the rare developmental condition dyskeratosis congenita, in which malignant transformation may occur.

Staphysagria (Staphisagria)

Homoeopathic stavesacre. A remedy for *craniomandibular dysfunction*, chronic *periodontitis* with a high *caries* rate, and *ranula*. It is especially indicated in those who suffer from stifled vexation and sexual repression, or those who have suffered sexual abuse. Also an important remedy for the control of pain and the promotion of healing in incisional wounds in relation to *oral surgery* in general, including periodontal surgery and apicectomy.

Stevens-Johnson syndrome – *see* Erythema multiforme

Sticta pulmonaria

Homoeopathic lung-wort. Used in the treatment of insomnia associated with *fractures*.

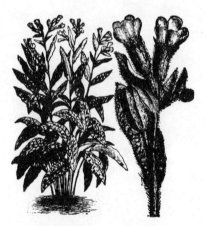

Fig. 42. Sticta pulmonaria

Stomatitis artefacta – *see* Cheek biting, recurrent

Stone – *see* Salivary calculus

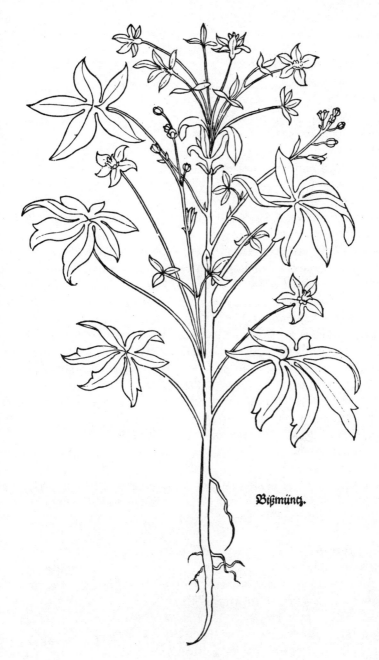

Fig. 43. Staphysagria

Strontium carbonicum

Homoeopathic strontium carbonate. A remedy for recurrent *dislocation* of the TMJ.

Subacute bacterial endocarditis, prevention of

Where appropriate antibiotics are unavailable, or where the patient refuses to take them, consider *Pyrogen* 30 twice daily, for one day prior to and seven days after the procedure.

See also *Amalgam, dental; Rheumatoid arthritis* (both with regard to bacterial antibiotic resistance).

Sulphur*

Homoeopathic sulphur. Used in the treatment of *aphthous ulcers, Behçet's disease,* delayed *eruption, angioedema, xerostomia, burning mouth syndrome, halitosis, herpes labialis,* atrophic *lichen planus, perioral dermatitis, mouth-breathing,* perversion of *taste* and *chickenpox*. A major constitutional remedy. **Susceptible typology:** may be thin or fat, red orifices, very philosophical, well-read, untidy, slovenly, dislike of bathing or washing, chilly in the day but hates hot rooms, hot at night and throws off bed-clothes, hunger at 11 am, thirsty, greedy, sweaty, itchy, ill-smelling, desires sweet things, desires fresh air, opens windows when others are chilly, burning pains, cannot stand still in one position, slouches or leans against something, early morning diarrhoea drives patient out of bed, periodicity and alternation of complaints, prone to skin diseases, prone to hypertension and haemorrhoids. A red centre with a red tip of the tongue tends to be indicative of its applicability.

Sulphur should always be used cautiously, since it tends to produce skin reactions in some patients, such as pruritis, pimples and boils. This is especially so in patients with a history of eczema, acne vulgaris, rosacea or boils. Should any reactions occur, it is prudent to discontinue the remedy and seek further advice.

Symphytum

Homoeopathic comfrey. The great remedy for the promotion of union of *fractures*. It will even treat non-union. It may also be used in *osteopetrosis* and *osteogenesis imperfecta*.

Syphilis

Associated with orogenital transmission, the primary lesion of this disease, a chancre, may be seen on the lip or oral mucosa. This is a nodule

Fig. 44. Symphytum

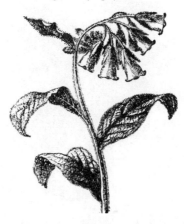

which breaks down to form an ulcer with indurated margins, and which, rather characteristically, is painless (unlike *herpes labialis*). The cervical lymph nodes have a rubbery consistency. This lesion generally resolves within 9 weeks, without scar formation. Secondary syphilis is a febrile illness, with generalised lymphadenopathy, a macular or papular rash, and the development of so-called snail track ulcers on the oral mucosa. Both primary and secondary lesions are highly infectious. Tertiary syphilis is unlikely to be seen these days, since most cases have been treated before this stage is entered. The characteristic intraoral features are the palatal gumma and syphilitic *leukoplakia* of the tongue, which latter is prone to malignant transformation. Any patient suspected of having syphilis should be urgently referred.

Syphilinum – *see* **Lueticum**

T

Taraxacum
Homoeopathic dandelion. Used in the treatment of *geographic tongue*. It is especially indicated in persons with cold finger-tips.

Tartar – *see* **Calculus, dental**

Taste, diminished or lost
Most cases of chronic and severe loss of taste and smell seem to result from a previous respiratory infection – either the common cold or

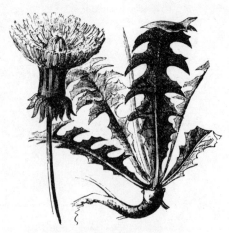

Fig. 45. Taraxacum

influenza. Many respond to *zinc* therapy, the usual adult dose being 30mg daily. This often requires administration for up to 18 months in order to rectify the problem, and lesser doses may be inadequate. Moderately diminished taste and smell is often associated with a chronic catarrhal state, which will require homoeopathic therapy. Loss of taste associated with a thick white or creamy coating on the tongue may indicate such remedies as *Antimonium crudum* and *Antimonium tartaricum*.

Taste, perversion of

Perversion of taste may occur spontaneously or in relation to specific foods. In a few cases, this is the result of offensive discharges from the sinuses or in relation to *gingivitis* or *periodontitis*. Gastric disease is another possible causative factor. Sometimes it arises from drug therapy. Electrochemical effects, resulting from the presence of dissimilar metals in the mouth, can produce spontaneous metallic tastes, which are only correctable by mechanical dental means. Many cases have no obvious causation. The homoeopathic materia medica abounds with remedies relating to perversion of taste. In order to be effective, a remedy should be selected upon the basis of both the susceptible typology and the individual character of the taste. As a generalisation, however, it may be said that certain remedies are very frequently indicated, viz. *Pulsatilla, Nux vomica, Mercurius solubilis* and *Sulphur*. *Natrum muriaticum* also deserves special attention with regard to a salty taste.

See also *Gonorrhoea; Rheumatoid arthritis* (with regard to penicillamine).

Tea tree oil (Oleum melaleucae)

Botanic. An oil obtained by distillation of the leaves of the Australian tea tree, Melaleuca alternifolia. It has antifungal and antibacterial properties, and is applied topically. It is useful in the treatment of oral *candidosis, angular cheilitis* and *herpes labialis*. It is either applied directly or in the form of a cream.

Teething, infant

Where the child is very fractious, with whining restlessness, wishing to be carried or petted, consider *Chamomilla* 30 1-hourly as necessary. This is the most commonly indicated remedy. Where the child is similar, but smells sour, consider *Rheum* 30 1-hourly as necessary. Where there is excessive salivation or halitosis, consider *Mercurius solubilis* 6 two or three times daily. Diarrhoea accompanying teething is not uncommon, and is covered by the three remedies mentioned. In the case of Rheum, the diarrhoea is also sour. *Podophyllum* is also occasionally useful in diarrhoea accompanying *eruption* of the teeth.

TMJ (Temporomandibular joint), disorders of

The majority of patients complaining of problems with the TMJ suffer from *craniomandibular dysfunction*. Sometimes the joint becomes a seat of inflammation in *rheumatoid arthritis*. Gout of the TMJ is extremely rare.

Less commonly, the joint itself has an isolated problem, such as a damaged meniscus. *Rhus toxicodendron* 30 two or three times daily is to be considered for uncomfortable but relatively painless cracking of the joint, which loosens with movement. Painful cracking of the joint indicates *Granatum* 6–30 two or three times daily. Pain in the joint upon swallowing suggests *Arum triphyllum* 30 two or three times daily.

See also *Dislocation, TMJ*.

Tension headache

These are seldom incapacitating, usually involve the occiput, may be unilateral or bilateral, and may spread to involve the whole head. Although many cases of so-called tension headache are ascribed to the psyche, the fact is that a large proportion suffer from vertebral subluxations in the cervicothoracic region of the spine. Tension headache should not be diagnosed until either *osteopathic* or *chiropractic* examination has been carried out, and any appropriate adjustments executed. *Acupuncture* may also be helpful. Some cases are also associated with *food allergy* or clinical hypoglycaemia. Either constitutional or *Bach flower remedies* may be indicated. Commonly indicated remedies include: *Gelsemium, Ignatia, Kali phosphoricum, Natrum carbonicum, Natrum muriaticum, Nux vomica, Podophyllum, Sepia* and *Spigelia*. Numerous other remedies may also be indicated, according to susceptible typology.

Tetanus

This serious infective disease often presents with jaw stiffness, which may be accompanied by neck stiffness, dysphagia and irritability. Any patient who presents with simple jaw stiffness, even without any companion symptoms, should be checked with regard to tetanus immunisation status. Should this be negative, and the person has received a wound of any sort, even the most minor puncture wound (as from a thorn), within the previous 15 weeks, or has been using unsterile hypodermic needles (as in drug abuse), then urgent referral is necessary.

See also *Trismus*.

Thalassaemia minor

A fairly common inherited disorder of haemoglobin synthesis producing mild *anaemia*, particularly in people of Mediterranean origin (e.g. those of Italian extraction). It may be confused with *iron* deficiency anaemia. Iron supplements should not be given for this disorder. Other more severe thalassaemia syndromes also exist.

Thiamine – *see* **Vitamin B1**

Thiosinaminum

Homoeopathic allyl sulphocarbamide (derived from mustard-seed oil). A remedy for the prevention and treatment of excessive *scar tissue*.

See also *Salivary glands, papillary or duct stricture of*.

Thrombocytopenia

An early sign of platelet deficiency may be the occurrence of petechiae in the oral mucosa, and observation of these should be regarded with suspicion. However, similar, but more transient lesions, may be seen in conjunction with the common *cold*, and about 30% of *glandular fever* cases exhibit petechiae. Thrombocytopenia is sometimes a manifestation of *AIDS*.

Thrush, oral – *see* **Candidosis, oral**

Thuja (Thuja occidentalis)

Homoeopathic arbor vitae. Thuja Ø must not be used in the mouth, either undiluted or diluted. A remedy for keloid *scar*, chronic *periodontitis*, predisposition to root *caries, epulis,* phenytoin *gingivitis, erythema multiforme, ranula, lymphangioma,* allergic *antibiotic* rash and human *papillomavirus lesions*. It may be indicated also in cases of trigeminal or glossopharyngeal *neuralgia*, particularly on the left side, and especially where the patient has the appropriate **susceptible typology:** overweight, < cold, < humidity, sensitive, impressionable, obsessional about minor matters, an oily face and dandruff, prone to polyps and warty growths, sweet or unpleasant sweat (droplets form on the upper lip), intolerant of onions.

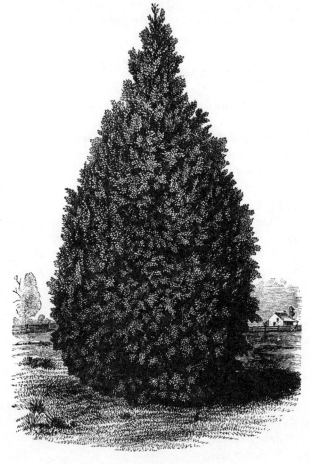

Fig. 46. Thuja

Thyropenia

A term which deserves resurrection. It may be taken to refer to those patients who exhibit the objective and subjective symptoms of *hypothyroidism*, yet are normal on routine testing for this disorder. In fact, many are borderline normal in tests, and suffer needlessly for years without proper treatment, which is identical to that for overt hypothyroidism.

Tic douloureux – *see* Neuralgia, trigeminal

Tic, neurotic facial

A repetitive spasm of facial muscles, occurring in neurotic persons or those under stress. Treatment generally involves homoeopathic constitutional treatment or *Bach flower remedies*.

Tick bites – *see* Lyme disease

Tocopherol – *see* Vitamin E

Tongue, bitten – *see* Bitten cheek or tongue

Tongue, black hairy (Lingua villosa)

This condition is characterised by elongation of the filiform papillae, and sometimes follows a course of antibiotics. The colour may actually vary from yellow-green, through brown to black. The condition may be asymptomatic, or may cause retching. Sometimes the tongue sticks to the roof of the mouth upon waking. Tongue-scraping or tongue-brushing is recommended. *Kali bichromicum* 6–30 three times daily may be helpful, together with *Myrrh* mouthwashes. Otherwise, either *Silicea* or *Natrum muriaticum* 6–30 twice daily may be considered, according to susceptible typology.

Tongue, burning – *see* Burning mouth syndrome

Tongue, fissured (Scrotal tongue)

Deep fissuring of the tongue is not uncommon, and may lead to irritation from stagnation of food in the crevices. Some cases seem to improve well with *vitamin B2* 50mg daily.

See also *Nitricum acidum*.

Tongue, geographic – *see* Geographic tongue

Tongue, indented
Those who are familiar with homoeopathy are aware that the presence of indentations of the teeth upon the tongue is regarded as a leader to the use of *Mercurius solubilis*. An indented tongue, however, is also a leader to over thirty other remedies, including *Arsenicum album, Calcarea carbonica, Iodum, Lueticum, Podophyllum, Pulsatilla, Rhus toxicodendron* and *Sepia*.

Tongue leaders
The tongue is not only an indicator of disease or deficiency, its appearance is also a leader to the prescription of many homoeopathic remedies. This subject is considered fully in 'Tongue that does not lie' by Prakash Vakil (2nd edition, 1988, Vakil Homoeopathic Prakashans).

See (for examples of homoeopathic leaders) *Bacillinum; Nitricum acidum; Nux vomica; Pulsatilla; Rhus toxicodendron; Sulphur; Tongue, indented*.

Tongue, scrotal – *see* Tongue, fissured

Tongue, sore – *see* Burning mouth syndrome

Tongue, varicose sublingual veins of
These tend to be indicative of the remedy *Nux vomica*.

Tooth-grinding & clenching – *see* Bruxism & bruxomania

Toothache
The weakness of the old homoeopathic authors was their inability to differentiate between different types of pathology, such as *pulpitis* and *pericoronitis*. These days, the selection of a simillimum is much easier, since the provision of a simple diagnostic label usually reduces the number of likely homoeopathic alternatives.

Toothpastes, homoeopathic & botanic
Various toothpastes are available containing botanic or potentised homoeopathic preparations, and generally lacking fluoride and peppermint. Botanic ingredients include *Krameria* and *Sanguinaria canadensis*. The absence of peppermint is said to be advantageous, in that this

substance is reputed to be antidotal to potentised homoeopathic remedies; either those which are normally prescribed or those contained within the toothpaste itself. In fact, clinical experience indicates that prescribed remedies are not antidoted by peppermint, provided that there is a minimal interval of approximately 10 minutes between the taking of a remedy and brushing the teeth.

See also *Fluoridation; Fluorosis.*

Torus mandibularis & palatinus

Both are *osteomata*, torus palatinus occurring in the midline of the hard palate, and torus mandibularis occurring on the lingual aspect of the pre-molar area of the mandible. These usually arise in adult life, treatment being by means of *oral surgery* or sometimes homoeopathy.

Traumatised tooth

Where the tooth is chipped and the dentine sensitive, get the patient to apply *Plantago Ø* three or four times daily (or more often, if necessary). Where the tooth exhibits mild pulpitic symptoms, give *Ferrum phosphoricum* 12–30 three times daily, a measure which may prevent pulpal necrosis. Where the pulp is actually exposed by dental fracture, give *Hypericum* 30–200 every 30 minutes or more, both before and after pulp-capping, until the pain is considerably reduced; thereafter proceed with Ferrum phosphoricum as described previously. Where the tooth has been loosened in its socket, give *Ruta* 6–30 three times daily, in addition to the other remedies mentioned. Further measures are required if either frank *pulpitis* or dental *abscess* occurs subsequently.

See also *Reimplantation.*

Trench mouth – see **Gingivitis, acute necrotising ulcerative**

Trigeminal neuralgia – see **Neuralgia, trigeminal**

Trismus (Locked jaw)

This is a concomitant of various oral conditions, including *craniomandibular dysfunction*, dental *abscess, pericoronitis, bruxism* and *dystonia*. Occasionally it is caused by drug therapies (phenothiazines), strychnine poisoning or *tetanus*. In all instances, the underlying cause must be treated or corrected. Additionally, *Cheiranthus* 30 two or three times daily is useful in benign cases. Trismus with shooting pains is sometimes better treated with *Hypericum* 30 three times daily.

Tropical sprue

This diarrhoeal disease may be acquired by exotic travellers. *Folate* deficiency is an important component. *Vitamin B12* and *iron* deficiencies may also be present. The oral mucosa becomes painful and red, and multiple *ulcers* develop.

Tuberculosis

Oral tuberculosis is relatively rare, but increasing numbers of cases are being seen as a complication of *AIDS*. Infection is usually secondary to pulmonary involvement. Any site in the mouth may be affected, but lesions occur more commonly on the tongue, hard and soft palates, and oropharynx. The lesions are nodules which break down to form painful irregular *ulcers* covered with a grey-white slough. Tuberculosis of the *salivary glands* is also occasionally seen.

The greatest risk to the dental surgeon, however, is pulmonary tuberculosis itself, even without oral manifestations. This is on the increase in major cities in the West, especially in Asian immigrant communities. The sputum of such patients is heavily infected.

Tumours & cysts

Malignancy should always be treated homoeopathically in conjunction with the recommendations of a cancer specialist.

Cysts and tumours causing expansion of the jaws may respond to *Hekla lava* 6 two or three times daily. In conjunction with *endodontic* technique, the use of this remedy may obviate the need for apicectomy in the case of a periapical cyst.

See also *Cistus canadensis; Fluorosis; Haemangioma; Kaposi's sarcoma; Mucocele; Osteoma; Pigmentation, oral & circumoral; Ranula; Salivary glands, neoplasms of.*

U

Ulcers (Ulceration) – *see* Agranulocytosis; AIDS; Allergy, orofacial; Angina bullosa haemorrhagica; Angular cheilitis; Aphthous ulcers *(common mouth ulcers);* Behçet's disease; Cancrum oris; Coeliac disease; Crohn's disease; Dermatitis herpetiformis; Epidermolysis bullosa; Erythema multiforme; Feverfew; Gingivitis, acute necrotising ulcerative; Gingivostomatitis, primary herpetic; Glandular fever;

Gonorrhoea; Granuloma inguinale; Hand, foot & mouth disease; Herpangina; Herpes labialis; Herpes zoster; Leishmaniasis; Leukaemia; Lichen planus; Linear IgA disease; Lip, median fissure of lower; Lymphogranuloma venereum; Median rhomboid glossitis; Necrotising sialometaplasia; Orofacial granulomatosis; Pemphigoid, mucous membrane; Pemphigus; Ramsay-Hunt syndrome; Reiter's syndrome; Rheumatoid arthritis; Syphilis; Tropical sprue; Tuberculosis; Tumours & cysts

V

Verbascum

Homoeopathic mullein. A remedy for trigeminal *neuralgia*. The pain affects the zygoma, *TMJ* and ear, especially on the left side, and is < talking, sneezing, the least movement, changes in temperature, and pressing the teeth together. Pains may occur twice daily, returning at the same hours of the morning and afternoon each day. A sensation as though the parts were crushed by tongs (or a similar device) is an important indication.

Verruca vulgaris

Common warts are sometimes seen on and around the lips of children. These are produced by human *papillomaviruses*. Some respond readily to *Thuja* 6–12 twice daily.

Vincent's stomatitis – see **Gingivitis, acute necrotising ulcerative**

Vitamin A

Deficiency may be involved in some cases of *periodontitis*. Overt symptoms of deficiency, such as night blindness and xerophthalmia (drying of the eye), may not be present. It is usefully given as cod-liver oil capsules, and is indicated in those who have a diet low in dairy products and margarines.

Vitamin B1 (Thiamine)

Deficiency of this vitamin is contributory to recurrent *aphthous* ulceration and *burning mouth syndrome* in some patients. Gross deficiency, which leads to beriberi, will not be seen by the average dental surgeon. Mild deficiency causes digestive disturbances, poor memory and concentration, loss of appetite, nausea, muscle weakness and fatigue. In therapy, 50–100mg daily may be given in adults.

Vitamin B2 (Riboflavine)

Deficiency may be implicated in some cases of oral *candidosis, burning mouth syndrome* and fissured *tongue*. It is frequently implicated in cases of *angular cheilitis*. Sore eyes, scaling of the skin (around the nose, mouth and forehead), and a magenta tongue are indicative of deficiency. In severe cases, a painful *glossitis* arises, initially pebbly in appearance (due to enlargement of the fungiform papillae), giving way to atrophy of the papillae and a smooth, shiny and fissured surface. In therapy, 50mg daily is a common adult dose.

Vitamin B6 (Pyridoxine)

Deficiency of this vitamin may be associated with some cases of recurrent *aphthous* ulceration and *burning mouth syndrome*. Therapy is especially indicated in women taking oral *contraceptives* or *hormone replacement therapy* (HRT), those on high protein diets, tobacco smokers, those who take alcohol regularly, and those on certain drugs, such as penicillamine. In therapy, 50mg three times daily may be given in adults, but this dose should not be exceeded.

See also *Carpal tunnel syndrome; Rheumatoid arthritis* (with regard to penicillamine).

Vitamin B12 (Hydroxocobalamin)

Deficiency may be associated with some cases of recurrent *aphthous* ulceration, *angular cheilitis, burning mouth syndrome* and oral *candidosis*. It is now thought that many vegetarians and vegans suffer from at least mild deficiency, and it has been suggested that they routinely take 100mcg daily by mouth. In therapy, for any of the previously mentioned conditions, this may be increased to 1000mcg daily.

Severe deficiency, which is usually associated with the inability to absorb the vitamin (but is not unknown in relation to veganism), produces pernicious anaemia. Fish tapeworm infestation, from eating raw or under-cooked fish (e.g. sushi), sometimes manifests itself similarly. The oral signs are a bright red, sore or burning, depapillated tongue and angular cheilitis. Unfortunately, many cases present merely with something resembling premature senility, unaccompanied by any other physical manifestations of deficiency. The problem is that the blood film can remain normal for a considerable period, whilst the tissues become slowly depleted of the vitamin. Severe cases of deficiency are treated by injection.

Vitamin B12, given by injection, may also be used in the treatment of *herpes zoster, herpes labialis,* post-herpetic *neuralgia* and *Ramsay-Hunt* syndrome.

See also *Crohn's disease; Folate; Tropical sprue.*

Vitamin C (Ascorbic acid)

Frank deficiency, resulting in scurvy, is unlikely to be seen. However, many people suffer from marginal deficiency, due to a diet deficient in fruit and vegetables. This may contribute to *gingivitis* and *periodontitis*. Poor wound healing in *oral surgery,* excessive *haemorrhage* and slow union of *fractures* may occur. Patients with a poor diet should take vitamin C 500mg twice daily by mouth. Given for some days prior to oral surgery, it may prevent some cases of excessive haemorrhage. Lack of vitamin C increases the predisposition to acquiring common infections, such as *colds and influenza.*

Vitamin D (Calciferol)

Gross deficiency, which leads to rickets or osteomalacia, is unlikely to be seen in developed countries. However, in those on a diet low in dairy products, margarines and oily fish, marginal deficiency may arise. Cod-liver oil is a good source of this vitamin.

See also *Calcium.*

Vitamin E (alpha – Tocopherol)

Deficiency may contribute to *gingivitis* and *periodontitis*. It is especially indicated in tobacco smokers, those with varicose veins or atherosclerosis, alcoholics, those with liver disease, those with an excessive intake of polyunsaturated fats, those who have had their gallbladders removed, and those with *coeliac disease* or cystic fibrosis. The usual adult therapeutic dose is 400–600IU daily (preferably as d-alpha tocopherol), but high doses such as these are not recommended in pregnancy. Vitamin E should not be given in cases of breast cancer. Vitamin E and *selenium* act synergistically.

Vitamin E is useful in the treatment of primary herpetic *gingivostomatitis*, *aphthous ulcers*, *herpes zoster* and post-herpetic *neuralgia*, *Ramsay-Hunt syndrome*, *burns*, *scalds* and keloid *scars*.

See also *Keratosis, smoker's*.

Voice, loss of – *see* **Laryngitis in dental surgeons**

von Willebrand's disease
An inherited disorder of blood clotting, which is usually mild in nature. Occasionally there is gingival bleeding from minimal trauma, and this may be confused with early *gingivitis*. It occurs in both men and women, and is extremely common. The bleeding tendency is characteristically aggravated by *aspirin*. There may be problems concerning *haemorrhage* in *oral surgery*, which should be carried out in a specialist centre.

W

Wisdom tooth, inflammation around – *see* **Pericoronitis**

Wrist, sprained
Take *Ruta* 12–30 three times daily, and apply *Arnica* Ø three or four times daily.

X

X-rays, ill-effects of – *see* **Radiography, ill-effects of**

Xerostomia
Dry mouth may be associated with *AIDS*, Sjögren's syndrome, radiotherapy or various drug treatments, including diuretics and psychogenic agents. Congential absence of one or more of the major salivary glands is a rare cause. Treatment of xerostomia in these cases will be determined by the cause, and may include the use of artificial saliva. Xerostomia of any origin increases the predisposition to oral *candidosis* and dental *caries*.

More commonly, however, xerostomia has no overt causation and must be considered to be constitutional. It is true to say that it occurs more frequently in those of an anxious nature. A remedy must be selected upon the basis of the mentals and generals of the case. The more commonly indicated remedies are *Aconite, Arsenicum album, Bryonia, Carbo vegetabilis, Ignatia, Kali bichromicum, Lachesis, Lycopodium, Natrum muriaticum, Nux vomica, Phosphorus, Pulsatilla, Rhus toxicodendron, Sepia, Silicea* and *Sulphur*.

Z

Zinc

Deficiency is extremely common. In fact, it is getting commoner as people incline towards vegetarianism, animal products being the best source of zinc. Overt signs are not always manifest. These include white spots on the nails, which break easily, and dryness of the skin and hair. Persons with zinc deficiency also tend to acquire infections more readily, such as *colds and influenza*, and *glandular fever*. They are also more easily fatigued. Zinc deficiency may be implicated in cases of recurrent *aphthous* ulceration, oral *candidosis, gingivitis, periodontitis* and *geographic tongue*. It is associated with poor healing of wounds and *fractures* in *oral surgery*. It is not uncommon in cases of *rheumatoid arthritis*. The usual therapeutic dose in adults is 15mg daily or 15mg twice daily (elemental zinc). Satisfactorily absorbed and cheap forms are chelated zinc and zinc citrate. Should *cramps* or itching occur, the dose must be reduced. Zinc *mouthwashes* are sometimes used in the treatment of periodontal disease.

Zincum metallicum

Homoeopathic metallic zinc. A remedy for *bruxism* or bruxomania in patients of appropriate typology. **Susceptible typology:** pale, emaciated tired, continual nervous movement of feet and legs, slowness of thought and comprehension from nervous fatigue, headaches < wine.

Zincum phosphoricum

Homoeopathic zinc phosphide. A remedy for *craniomandibular dysfunction*, where there are sharp pains of the head and face, especially in nervously exhausted patients (students, businessmen, professionals, etc.).

Zingiber

Botanic. Common ginger root. Zingiber Ø is useful in the treatment of *colds and influenza*. It also prevents and treats travel-sickness. Should a child (or adult) arrive in the surgery with this complaint, give 1 drop per 10kg of body weight in a teaspoonful of water.

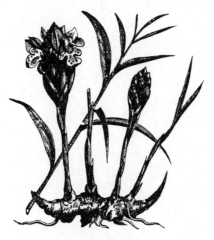

Fig. 47. Zingiber

APPENDIX ONE

The Basic Dental Pharmacy

The following is a list of useful remedies, other substances, and optional sundries to be stocked by the dental surgeon. Others may be added at leisure and according to demand and experience.

Simples

Aconite 30, pilules 7g
Amalgam (dental) 30, pilules 7g
Argentum nitricum 30, pilules 7g
Arnica 30, pilules 7g, liquid potency 10ml
Arsenicum album 30, pilules 7g
Belladonna 30, pilules 7g
Borax 30, pilules 7g
Calendula Ø, 30ml
Calendula 5% ointment, 50g
Carbo vegetabilis 30, liquid potency 5ml
Chamomilla 30, pilules 7g, liquid potency 10ml
Cheiranthus 30, pilules 7g
Coccus cacti 30, pilules 7g
Coffea cruda 30, pilules 7g
Ferrum phosphoricum 30, pilules 7g
Feverfew 30, pilules 7g
Gelsemium 30, pilules 7g
Hepar sulph. 6, pilules 7g

Hepar sulph. 30, pilules 7g
Hypericum 30, pilules 7g
Ignatia 30, pilules 7g
Lachesis 30 pilules 7g
Ledum 30, pilules 7g
Mercurius solubilis 30, pilules 7g
Myrrh Ø, 30ml
Myristica 30, pilules 7g
Phosphorus 30, pilules 7g
Plantago Ø, 30ml
Propolis Ø, 30ml
Pyrogen 30, pilules 7g
Rhus toxicodendron 30, pilules 7g
Ruta 30, pilules 7g
Silicea 6, pilules 7g
Staphysagria 30, pilules 7g

Mixtures
China 6/Phosphorus 12/Ferrum phosphoricum 30, liquid potency 10ml
Ipecacuanha 30/Millefolium 30, liquid potency 10ml
Rescue remedy, 10ml
Smelling salts, 17ml bottle

Supplements
Coenzyme Q10 30mg, 60 capsules
Vitamin B2 50mg, 100 capsules
Vitamin C 500mg, 100 tablets
Vitamin E (d-alpha tocopherol) 600IU, 60 capsules
Zinc 15mg (chelate/citrate), 100 tablets/capsules

Sundries
Amber dispensing vials (plastic or glass) 10–15ml, 50
Amber glass bottles 50ml, 30
Personalized labels, bearing your name, qualifications, address, telephone number and the warning 'Keep out of the reach of children'

Suppliers
The following are postal suppliers, who also stock relevant books or pamphlets:

Ainsworth's Homoeopathic Pharmacy
36 New Cavendish Street
London W1M 7LH, England
Tel: 0171 935 5330

Brauer Biotherapies
1 Para Road
PO Box 234
Tanunda
South Australia 5352
Tel: 085 63 2932

Lamberts Healthcare Ltd.
1 Lamberts Road
Tunbridge Wells TN2 3EQ, England
Tel: 01892 552120/552121
(suppliers of excellent nutritional supplements only)

Nelson's Homoeopathic Pharmacy
73 Duke Street
London W1M 6BY, England
Tel: 0171 629 3118

Standard Homeopathic
210 West 131st Street
Box 61067
Los Angeles
California 90061, USA
Tel: 800 624 9659

Weleda (UK) Ltd.
Heanor Road
Ilkeston
Derbyshire, DE7 8DR, England
Tel: 01602 309319

Since area dialling codes change occasionally, please check with the operator if you cannot obtain the appropriate number.

APPENDIX TWO

Mercury Toxicity

contributed by
Catherine Price, BDS
Secretary BHDA, Membership Secretary IAOMT (UK)

& edited by
Dr Colin B. Lessell

In 1818, a British chemist, Bell, discovered that, by mixing silver fragments obtained from filing silver coins with mercury, he could make a paste, which could be shaped before it set into a hard metal alloy. In 1826, a French dentist began applying the amalgam for the purpose of filling teeth.

By 1830, this new material also contained tin and copper, and was being used to fill dental cavities in North America, the advisability and safety of which had already become a matter of great controversy. The Victorians were well aware of the symptoms of mercury poisoning, if only from its widespread use in the hatting industry. The phrase, which has become part of the English language, 'as mad as a hatter', and the well-known Mad Hatter of Alice in Wonderland, published in 1897, are familiar examples of the insanity and mental derangements associated with mercury vapour. Furthermore, the widely practised art of fire-gilding of bronze to produce ormolu resulted in the same fate for the artisan.

In 1840, the American Society of Dental Surgeons debarred its members from using the new mercury amalgam, subsequently suspending several New York City dentists in 1848 for 'malpractice for using mercury fillings'. Nonetheless, the great advantages of this cheap and easily used material led to the formation of a new dental group in 1859, which is now the American Dental Association. It is worthy of note that, at the time of publication of the present textbook, both the American and British Dental Associations still advocate that the use of mercury amalgam is good and safe in practice!

Thus, conservative dentistry was made available to the masses when, hitherto, only the wealthy could aspire to the alternative gold restorations.

The mercury amalgams currently available vary in their constitutent parts, but a typical composition is: mercury 50%, silver 35%, tin 13% and copper 2%. Zinc is often present as a trace element. A large filling can contain as much as 1g of mercury.

Until recent years, the official position has been that the mercury contained within an amalgam filling cannot escape after the material has hardened. Unfortunately for officialdom, and more so for the patient, the converse has been indisputably demonstrated. Mercury vapour escapes from amalgam restorations in measurable and significant quantities, both in the passive and the active situations. Moreover, the degree of loss associated with mastication or bruxism is much higher. It has been estimated that a non-bruxist with eight occlusal fillings can release as much as 300mcg daily. A bruxist can release amounts dangerously approaching industrial levels!

The World Health Organisation (WHO) document 'Environmental Health Criteria 118', concerning inorganic mercury, states that the largest estimated daily intake and retention of mercury and mercury compounds in the general public, not occupationally exposed, is from dental amalgams. WHO has stated that *there is no safe dose of mercury*. Mercury is a poison at any level, whether or not the level of intoxication is sufficient to produce recognisable symptoms.

Two levels of mercury poisoning are recognised. *Acute mercurialism* is a condition which develops from a single and significant exposure to mercury, such as that associated with the fracture of a thermometer or surgery spillage. Its symptoms include: a harsh and metallic taste; burning pains in the mouth, throat and stomach; profuse salivation; abdominal pains; diarrhoea and vomiting. *Chronic mercurialism* is more insidious in onset, and has a range of symptoms, the significance of which may be readily misdiagnosed. These include: psychological disturbances; irritability and outbursts of anger; nervousness; loss of memory; inability to concentrate; and depressive states.

In the absence of any scientific evidence that mercury is actually beneficial (of which there is none to date), we shall restrict ourselves to a consideration of a few of the more notable pieces of research that relate to mercury toxicity:

(1) *The spread of radioactively labelled mercury from amalgam in sheep teeth to mother and foetus after 16, 33 and 73 days.* Vimy et al. University of Calgary. American Journal of Physiology, 258, 1990.

In this study, radioactively tagged mercury, of a type not naturally found, was mixed into a dental amalgam. This was then placed in the teeth of sheep. At the end of the period of study, radiographs demonstrated concentrations of the tagged mercury in the kidneys, brains, livers, thyroids and pituitary glands of both the ewe and the unborn foetus. Deposition was also observed in the placenta. Furthermore, there was radiographic evidence of large concentrations in the jaws, despite the fact that all the filled teeth had been subsequently extracted.

(2) *Mercury from dental 'silver' tooth fillings impairs sheep kidney function.* Boyd, Benediktsson, Vimy & Lorscheider. University of Calgary, 1991.

In this study, mercury amalgam fillings were inserted into the teeth of adult ewes, whilst control ewes were given glass ionomer fillings. Renal function was evaluated before the placement of the fillings, and at 30 and 60 days afterwards. The inulin clearance rate in the non-control group diminished dramatically, and by 60 days they all showed a 60% reduction and a substantially lowered renal filtration rate (33–89%). It was concluded that mercury from amalgams has the capacity to reduce renal function.

(3) *Mercury released from 'silver' fillings provokes an increase in mercury and antibiotic resistant bacteria in the primate oral and intestinal flora.* Summers, Wireman, Vimy, Lorscheider, Marshall, Levy, Bennett and Billard. University of Calgary. Antimicrobial Agents and Chemotherapy, 37, 1993.

Most bacteria cannot survive in the presence of mercury, but those which continue to exist do so by acquiring a genetic resistance to the toxic effects of that substance.

In an investigation of 640 human subjects, with regard to a sub-group of 356 persons with no recent exposure to antibiotics, it was demonstrated that those with a high prevalence of mercury-resistance in their intestinal bacteria were significantly more likely to have bacteria resistant to two or more antibiotics.

In a follow-up study using monkeys, each of which received 16 occlusal amalgam fillings, a large proportion of their common oral and intestinal bacteria became resistant to mercury within 2 weeks of placement of amalgam fillings. Of particular significance is the fact that nearly all of the mercury resistant strains from these monkeys were also resistant to one or more antibiotics, including ampicillin, chloramphenicol, tetracycline and streptomycin; despite the fact that these monkeys had not been exposed to antibiotics. From 12–50% of the multi-resistant bacteria examined could transfer their resistance to an antibiotic-sensitive laboratory strain. In two of the three studies, the amalgam fillings were replaced with non-mercuric composite resin fillings; after which, the proportion of mercury and antibiotic resistant bacterial populations declined during the subsequent 2 months.

It was concluded that, since dental amalgam is the greater source of mercury exposure for humans, other than occupational exposure, it is likely that dental amalgam mercury is a selective agent which increases the prevalence of plasmid-associated mercury and antibiotic resistances in the oral and intestinal flora of humans. That such resistant plasmids can compromise the efficacy of antibiotics used in the treatment of bacterial infections is well documented. Further studies in this are continuing.

A study has been published which shows that there is a statistically significant correlation between the number of human occlusal surfaces filled with mercury amalgam and the levels of mercury detectable in the blood, measurable in nanograms per ml. Even such tiny levels may be of some significance in sensitive individuals.

Dr Gustav Drasch, a forensic toxicologist at the University of Munich, has shown that mercury, as is the case with sheep, crosses the human placental barrier. Amongst his findings is the fact that the mercury levels in foetal kidneys and livers, and the levels in the kidneys and cerebral cortices of babies aged 10–50 weeks, are statistically related to the numbers of maternal amalgam fillings.

Ongoing research being performed by Dr Boyd Haley at the University of Kentucky, USA, suggests, from autopsy results, that the mercury from dental amalgam may be implicated in Alzheimer's disease. Many feel that this disorder is produced by a combination of toxicity and deficiency, and thus may be preventable in the future.

In summary

(1) Mercury is acknowledged to be a powerful toxic agent, for which WHO cannot state a safe level.

(2) It is widely acknowledged that mercury vapour escapes from dental amalgam restorations.

(3) Eating hot foods, mastication and bruxism drastically increase the levels of mercury release.

(4) The vapour is inhaled, ingested and absorbed through the oral mucosa and lungs, and passes into the bloodstream.

(5) Scientific research has shown that mercury lodges in the brain, heart, lungs, liver, kidneys, thyroid, pituitary, adrenals and red blood cells. It suppresses the immune system. Mercury also crosses through the placenta, whence it lodges in similar sites in the unborn foetus. It has been shown to be present in breast milk in higher concentrations than in the blood.

(6) There is a correlation between the number of tooth surfaces filled with amalgam and the levels of mercury in the brain. There is a further correlation between brain mercury levels and Alzheimer's disease.

(7) Mercury induces normal oral and intestinal bacteria to become resistant to antibiotics.

Protocols For The Safe Removal Of Amalgam Fillings

Thus far, all the discussion has been with the emphasis upon the potential risks to the patient. It should not be forgotten that the dental team is also at risk from occupational exposure to mercury vapour produced in the practice of placing and removing amalgam fillings. As early as 1926, the German chemist, Dr. Alfred Stock, researched mercury poisoning and identified the fact that amalgam restorations were a source of mercury vapour.

The dentist should be aware of the fact that it is becoming increasingly common for employees to seek compensation for damage to health sustained in the workplace. As long as there are patients requiring old amalgam fillings to be replaced, there will be an inevitable exposure of the dental team to mercury vapour. Every effort should be made to reduce the levels of exposure to an absolute minimum. In this respect, we must consider the health of all the workers within the practice, from the dentist to the cleaner.

The International Academy of Oral Medicine and Toxicology (IAOMT) has established a recommended protocol for the safer removal of mercury amalgam fillings and the subsequent disposal of waste. IAOMT seeks to educate the dental profession and to encourage a changeover to the use of the most biocompatible materials available, as well as to stimulate and fund relevant research programmes.

Absorption of mercury vapour from occupational exposure is primarily through the lungs, with a much lesser degree of absorption occuring through the skin, via droplets or dust. The absorbed mercury is then distributed throughout the body and is stored in various organs, including the brain. Research published in 1989 suggests that mercury vapour is able to travel from the nasopharynx to the floor of the cranial cavity, where it becomes concentrated in the pituitary gland. The pathway is thought to be via the olfactory nerves or the cranial venous system, both of which routes bypass the liver, which is the main detoxifying organ of the body. From autopsy studies of pituitary glands taken from Swedish dentists, it was demonstrated that the level of mercury in those glands was, on average, 2.5 times higher than that found in the cerebral cortex. In one case, the level was 169 times higher!

The half-life of mercury in the bloodstream is estimated to be 3 days; yet, once absorbed into body tissues, this is extended to 90 days. Mercury compounds bind to body tissues by virtue of their affinity for thiol (–SH) chemical groups. These are found in all enzymes and most proteins. By acting as non-specific enzyme inhibitors, mercury compounds are able to affect membrane permeability, the conduction of nerve impulses and tissue respiration. The biochemical effects have been compared with those of the venom of the black widow spider (*Latrodectus spp.*).

The body excretes mercury mainly in the urine and faeces; the latter in such high concentrations that raw sewage is considered by the Swedes to be toxic waste on environmental grounds.

Clearly, the key areas upon which to focus attention are:

(1) The elimination of risk of inhalation of mercury vapour.

(2) The prevention of skin contamination from dust and droplets of the aerosol created by high-speed turbines.

(3) Taking measures to 'mop up' mercury compounds from the blood.

(4) Taking measures to encourage the expulsion of long-standing accumulated mercury compounds from the body tissue.

Recommended protocol for the benefit of the dental team

Ideally, the treatment room should have an in-built air filtration system, with specific mercury filters to eliminate the concentration of mercury vapour levels in the room air. There should also be a floor-level mercury filter, since mercury vapour is heavier than air and thus sinks to the floor. It follows that personnel should avoid wearing open-toed shoes, and that trousers should be worn by all staff.

Both the dentist and assistant should wear some form of mercury filtration mask and a full-face visor to protect the skin and eyes from aerosol contamination. The mercury mask and visor can be removed once amalgam removal is completed.

Ideally, an impermeable protective cape should be worn during the amalgam removal process, and it has been suggested that gloves worn whilst removing the fillings should be discarded, and the hands washed before re-gloving. This is because some researchers have demonstrated that mercury vapour passes through the gloves and accumulates next to the skin. Impermeable hair coverings should also be worn.

Copious amounts of water coolant spray should be used, in that the mercury vapour pressure doubles with every 10°C rise in temperature. Tungsten carbide, rather than diamond, burrs should be used in order to facilitate sectioning of the amalgam into large portions; thus reducing slurry formation and associated extra vapour.

The use of a high volume aspiration system is essential, and special suction tips are now readily available, which maximise vapour removal. Some workers believe that the use of dental dam is unessential if such tips are used. The suction and drainage systems should have mercury extraction filters incorporated, in order to prevent noxious emissions into the environment. Waste particles collected from the filtration systems should be properly stored in sealed containers supplied for this purpose, and ultimately disposed of as toxic waste.

Appropriate nutritional support, prescribed on the basis of sound scientific testing, may be necessary, and such prescriptions should be properly monitored. Suggested supplementation protocols are obtainable from IAOMT and BHDA.

Recommended protocol for the benefit of the patient

The patient should be ideally draped in an impermeable cape for the removal of amalgam restorations. Some workers also advocate the provision of an impermeable hair covering.

The homoeopathic remedy *Mercurius solubilis* 6, taken twice daily, is often used for the entire period of treatment, in order to oppose mercury toxicity. An alternative is homoeopathic amalgam. *Amalgam* 30c is taken twice daily on the day preceding, the day of, and the day following an appointment for amalgam removal. It is sensible to have taken charcoal by mouth prior to the appointment, in order to absorb any mercury entering the stomach or intestines. It is prudent to point out, however, that charcoal may have the effect of reducing the efficacy of oral contraceptives, and also that many available charcoal preparations are encapsulated in gelatin, thus being objectionable to true vegetarians, vegans and many Hindus.

The eyes should be covered with a simple dampened gauze, protective wrap-around spectacles or special spectacles which send a constant flow of air across the eyes, in order to dispel vapour.

Many workers still advocate the use of a dental dam; although there is some evidence that mercury vapour may pass straight through it, or via imperfections of seal, and accumulate in high concentration beneath the dam itself. There are many other advantages in the use of the dental dam, besides protection from mercury vapour, and these need to be considered before a decision is made (always with the informed consent of the patient).

A nose-piece delivering air can be used, or a simple mercury vapour mask. If the dam covers the nose, it is questionable whether such a precaution is necessary.

After the amalgam filling is removed, the protective clothing can be discarded, and the patient should wipe his/her face with a hot towel before continuing with the restorative phase of the appointment.

Mercury Levels & Chelation
Accurate biochemical testing for chronic mercurialism is very difficult to achieve. Tissue sampling is not appropriate, and X-ray fluorescence is not widely available. Analysis is restricted to a limited range of biological samples, and the results thus obtained are not always reliable. Blood mercury levels do not reflect the amount absorbed by body tissues, and the half-life of 3 days means that an isolated blood sample may not necessarily give an accurate representation of periodic exposure.

Hair and finger-nail analysis provide quite good indications of exposure to organic mercury compounds, such as methyl and ethyl mercury, but inorganic mercury (such as that from amalgam) is insufficiently accumulated in these tissues to form the basis of reliable results.

The mercury levels in urine can accurately reflect the total body burden. However, there are difficulties in testing urine for mercury. The tests should be performed over a 24 hour period, in order to allow for fluctuations of urinary output. If a single specimen is to be used, the test result must be related to the creatinine level. This is a waste product of muscle metabolism, and is used clinically as an index of glomerular filtration rate.

Recent developments at the time of writing have suggested that a very accurate analysis, called the PIXE test, enables X-irradiated blood samples to be examined microscopically to demonstrate sites on the red blood corpuscles occupied by mercury.

Certain chelating agents, such as DMSA (Dimercaprol succinic acid) and DMPS (2, 3, Dimercapto-propane-1-sulphonate), given under medical supervision, are useful in ridding the body of its accumulated mercury.

Epilogue

With countries such as Sweden working towards a total ban on the use of mercury amalgam (upon environmental grounds), the dental profession, as providers of health care, need to equip themselves with the knowledge, materials and expertise, not only to remove amalgam fillings with safety, but also to replace them with the most biocompatible restorations available.

This requires a constant and ongoing quest for knowledge and information; and an ability and willingness to change practising habits and techniques which become obsolescent. It is important not to have a closed mind, with inflexible viewpoints and resistance to change.

It is important to have a mind that is open; but not at both ends, so that everything falls out!

Editorial comment

Mercury is a substance of well-documented and established toxicity. Even before the more recent studies concerning the release of mercury vapour from dental amalgams, this had been firmly established. The opponents to the mercury issue state that it is unrealistic to insert multiple amalgams in the teeth of herbivores (viz. sheep), who, by their very nature, chew for considerable periods of time, and deduce from the results a supposed significant vapour release in the human situation. Even accepting this argument, mercury in the dental surgery, at the time of amalgam preparation and placement, constitutes a formidable and undeniable hazard to the patient, operator, assistants and the environment. Upon this basis alone, there is no sensible reason, other than that of pure economics, to continue with the provision of amalgam restorations. It follows, therefore, that all broken or lost fillings should be replaced with non-mercuric materials; since, although there may be some potentially toxic substances released from them, their toxicity has never been properly demonstrated, as is the case with mercury itself. It would thus be a sign of lunacy to consider any other recourse.

We must now pass to the more tricky matter of sound amalgam restorations already *in situ*, and whether they should be routinely removed. My own view is that they should not, unless there is good reason to suspect that they are actually causing harm. Their removal alone, by releasing significant quantities of mercury vapour, is hazardous to the patient, operator, assistants and environment. Bruxists will receive some reasonable protection by the wearing of acrylic splints at night.

The determination of whether existing amalgam restorations are harmful to the patient, apart from the more obvious sign of lichenoid reactions, is, however, difficult. Assessment of mercury levels in the body may be helpful in this respect, but it must not be forgotten that people vary considerably in their sensitivity to toxins. Whilst it is possible to make the general statement that there is no determinable safe level of mercury, certain individuals are surprisingly resistant to toxic action. For example, the recent increase in adult asthma in the UK has been attributed to environmental pollution; yet this does not affect all individuals equally, and many show no obvious ill-effects at all. Rasputin could not be poisoned with arsenic, since, it is alleged, he took small quantities of that substance throughout his life. Some humans, rather like some bacteria, are incredibly adaptive to toxic environments.

Where the patient presents with a certain set of symptoms, and these cannot be attributed to any other cause, it is not unreasonable to consider amalgam removal, provided that those symptoms are consistent with our present knowledge of chronic mercurialism. There can, for example, be a close correspondence between the symptoms of ME (postviral syndrome) and those of chronic mercury intoxication. Many such cases respond well to nutritional and homoeopathic therapies. Amalgam removal should only be considered as an ultimate resort in unresponsive cases, and not as a primary therapy.

Suggested reading
Dentistry without Mercury. Dr Sam F. Ziff (ISBN 0–941011–04–6).
Mercury Exposure Hazards and Risk Management, A Manual for the Dental Practitioner. Stephen Hewitt (ISBN 1–874692–00–9).

Useful addresses
IAOMT (UK), 72 Harley Street, London W1N 1AE, England.
BHDA, c/o The Faculty of Homoeopathy, The Royal London Homoeopathic Hospital, Great Ormond Street, London WC1N 3HR, England.

Index

Italicised topics indicate homoeopathic or botanic medicines. Italicised numerals indicate principal entries.